FORGETTING
ITEMS

FORGETTING ITEMS

The Social Experience of Alzheimer's Disease

Baptiste Brossard

INDIANA UNIVERSITY PRESS

This book is a publication of

Indiana University Press
Office of Scholarly Publishing
Herman B Wells Library 350
1320 East 10th Street
Bloomington, Indiana 47405 USA

iupress.indiana.edu

Manufactured in the United States of America

Library of Congress Cataloging-in-Publication Data

Names: Brossard, Baptiste, 1985- author.
Title: Forgetting items : the social experience of
Alzheimer's disease / Baptiste Brossard.
Other titles: Oublier des choses. English
Description: Bloomington, Indiana : Indiana University Press, 2019. |
Translation of Oublier des choses : ce que vivent les
malades d'Alzheimer / Baptiste Brossard. 2017. |
Includes bibliographical references and index.
Identifiers: LCCN 2019017258 (print) | LCCN 2019018527 (ebook) |
ISBN 9780253044990 (ebook) | ISBN 9780253044969
(hardback : alk. paper) |
ISBN 9780253044983 (pbk. : alk. paper)
Subjects: | MESH: Alzheimer Disease—psychology |
Interpersonal Relations | Caregivers
Classification: LCC RC523 (ebook) |
LCC RC523 (print) | NLM WT 161 | DDC 616.8/311—dc23
LC record available at https://lccn.loc.gov/2019017258

1 2 3 4 5   24 23 22 21 20 19

CONTENTS

Acknowledgments   *vii*

Introduction   *ix*

1   The Organization of Repairing Exchanges   *1*

2   Losing Credibility   *35*

3   The Deference Industry   *71*

4   Reconstituting People   *101*

   Conclusion   *127*

Notes   *135*

Index   *147*

ACKNOWLEDGMENTS

Some fieldwork studies on which this book relies have been realized with the collaboration of Solène Billaud, Normand Carpentier, and Pamela Skaff. This work has been supported by two funding sources: la Fondation Plan Alzheimer (France, 2012–2014) and le partenariat ARIMA (Québec, 2014–2016). The translation is by Baptiste Brossard and Rohan Todd.

The author wishes to thank, in particular, all the participants who accepted to meet with him and give him time either at difficult moment of their lives or when time was a rare commodity.

INTRODUCTION

"CARS ARE RUSHING IN ALL DIRECTIONS; PEDESTRIANS AND cyclists are trying to thread their way through the mêlée of cars; policemen stand at the main crossroads to regulate the traffic with varying success. But this external control is founded on the assumption that every individual is himself regulating his behavior with the utmost exactitude in accordance with the necessities of this network. The chief danger that people here represent for others results from someone in this bustle losing his self-control."[1]

In his book *State Formation and Civilization*, the sociologist Norbert Elias uses urban circulation as an illustration of the strict control that individuals must impose on themselves in contemporary societies in order not to disturb the public order. Everyone contributes to the organization of social life—chaotic in appearance yet ordered in reality—by remaining focused, self-controlled, and aware of the multiple rules that govern us. We comport ourselves in line with some norms and configure our emotions in the image of those supposedly deemed appropriate. The ability to self-control is a fundamental feature of contemporary social life, the exercising of which remains inseparable from deep cultural expectations shaped by economic imperatives, themselves grounded in presumptions about individual "autonomy." The extent to which such "autonomy" is celebrated in our societies is evident in the way that we often regard the imposition of such constraints as fruits of our own individuality, as if controlling ourselves is simply a raw manifestation of our free will.

It is only when one of the elements of this imperative to self-control seems to falter—that is, when one no longer adheres to dominant norms and accepted emotional configurations—that one can observe the extent to which this order, seemingly "natural" at first sight, is in fact socially maintained.

This is the case with people diagnosed with Alzheimer's disease or other forms of dementia—I will employ these two expressions as equivalent to facilitate the development of this book. Patients suffering from dementia/Alzheimer's undermine the foundations of public order, grounded as it is on the individual's ability to act as an autonomous and conditioned agent. Around those affected by dementia, a set of interactions and devices begins to emerge that frames the sufferer's trouble and prevents them from too much "damage" to bodies and interactions.

Therefore, the study I propose is less a study of a health condition than an exploration of the general "interaction order" through one of its possible systematic alterations: dementia. How do these interactions occur? What do they produce? What does this production tell us about our social world?

Beyond the Medical Discourse

According to the World Alzheimer's Association, in 2016 there were 47.5 million people diagnosed with Alzheimer's disease. The scale of this disease is arguably one of the most serious public health problems of our time.

In the West, the origins of Alzheimer's and other illnesses that impair the "normal" functioning of memory and thinking are attributed to some dysfunction of the brain. Such dysfunction is often characterized by amyloid plaques that form in most patients or else to some dysfunction of the body more generally, since certain lifestyles would favor the onset of the disease. Given that Alzheimer's disease is conventionally understood in these ways, the dominant field of expertise is medical.[2] This means that doctors figure as the most legitimate actors to discuss the behaviors and interactions associated with dementia.

Furthermore, this is why many books (especially outside the social sciences) that deal with dementia are based on the medical representation of health problems. This medical representation entails a clinical depiction of the symptoms and their progression through stages, which is associated with the possible causes of the illness and some indications regarding what needs to be done in terms of treatment. These indications often accompany some rather vague ethical recommendations, such as invitations to behave with "humanity," "decency," or "respect" and to support the "dignity" of the patients. This discourse generates such a consensus that one may wonder what a sociologist could possibly add.

What if we were to apprehend Alzheimer's disease through the interactions that *make it* on a regular basis? What if we focus on the ways of acting, behaving, and framing the symptoms, all the elements that construct the disease in its daily reality, both for patients and people around them? What if we focus on the *social experience of dementia*?

Methodology: Investigating an Interaction Network

[The geriatrist looks at the sheets on his desk and takes a serious tone].
  "Well, in terms of . . . of all that we've seen . . . the tests, the MRI . . . I would say . . . that it's most likely Alzheimer's. It's clear that there are some obvious memory problems. So, I'll give you a prescription and we'll see you in six months."
  Silence in the room.

I started this work in October 2011, in Paris, attending seventy consultations devoted to the diagnosis of dementia. Initially wanting to study medical diagnostic techniques, I understood that Alzheimer's disease "is" also a relational mechanism. A mechanism in which patients play, and often lose, their *credibility* toward health professionals and their relatives, who no longer believe what they say. During interviews conducted with some patients, I was struck by the relational reconfigurations taking place around them in a situation of indefinite waiting: "We'll see," a lady repeated nervously, "we'll see." In the five following years, I conducted various fieldwork studies in order to explore what dementia implies in various places and for different people.[3]

Between summer 2012 and summer 2013, I studied how the medical profession builds and adopts diagnostic tools. In particular, I focused on the mini-mental state examination, a neuropsychological test used throughout the world. Moreover, together with my colleague Solène Billaud, I embarked on an in-depth study of Mr. Lautrec's diary. Mr. Lautrec is an octogenarian suspected by his relatives to be suffering from cognitive disorders and placed against his will in a nursing home. His family suspects him of being paranoid because he reports everything that happens to him in his notebook. Mr. Lautrec's family consider that such a practice is symptomatic of cognitive disorder. It seemed, however, in a context where Mr. Lautrec was receiving an array of medical services, in part against his will, writing had become a vital organizational activity. That is, we recognized that symptoms cannot be isolated from the situation in which the persons are, from their social, historical context.[4]

In the fall of 2013, I decided to study nursing homes more specifically because many people diagnosed with dementia end up in nursing homes or aged-care facilities. I was intrigued as to what changes such institutionalization implies. For six months, I spent two or three days a week observing the collective life of residents in a private institution in the Paris region, which contains two closed units welcoming people with severe cognitive disorders.[5] When the occasion permitted, I also conducted interviews with the residents. I was particularly interested in the interactions between staff members and residents. A typical example of such interactions follows:

> [A staff member serves a glass of water to a resident] "Here it is, Miss Henriquez. Is it okay like that?"
> [The resident bows her head] "Oh . . ."
> "You'll see your daughter soon, yeah? Is she coming tomorrow?"
> "I dunno . . ."

These multiple "little gestures" ultimately build up institutional life and shape the ways in which residents perceive and experience it. Arriving in Montreal in July 2014, I continued my work on nursing homes. However, I now wanted to know the backstage, the set of interactions and constraints underlying those gestures. I met about twenty nursing aides[6] willing to partake in interviews with me. These nursing aides are the professionals most in touch with the residents and their daily lives. They told me about their strategies of everyday "tinkering" to cope with various situations. They spoke of ways to "tinker" with uncooperative residents who do not want to take their bath or to eat, and in other cases they spoke of strategies with which to approach residents with whom no contact seems possible. In the nursing home, everything is a matter of attention, of diversions, of "little gestures."

However, we should not forget that beyond the nursing aides, an entire organization works toward producing these interactions. Thus, alongside my observations of institutional life and interviews with nursing aides, I observed two unit managers in nursing homes, this time in the public sector, for a period of ten days each. To run their units, these executives interact with a range of actors, from nurses to branch employees, in a range of different contexts, from formal meetings to casual talks in the corridors. As we move up the professional hierarchy, it is also necessary to take into consideration all of the accreditations that the health facilities must obtain in order to gain their right to exercise treatment and care. There are hundreds of standards to be followed in the Canadian context. Accreditation Canada, an independent organization specializing in health services, and the Quebec Department of Health and Social Services are the organizing bodies that preside over the accreditation process. I was able to develop a multilayered picture of institutional life on the basis of discussions with the managers responsible for upholding institutional norms and the study of the documents produced over the course of our discussions. I was able to perceive, in particular, how words coming from "above" convert into interactions with the residents, each interpreted at different levels of the hierarchy.

For two years, I also worked with Normand Carpentier, a Canadian sociologist who has done extensive work with caregivers in institutional settings. For ten years Normand and his team conducted an interview every two years with sixty family caregivers in the Montreal region. This opportunity to analyze these stories provided me with a long-term follow-up of the information quests, hesitations, and changing power relationships experienced by patients and their families during the course of the illness, from the first disorders to the eventual placement in an institution. Again,

I observed how the development of symptoms interweaves with the familial, medical, and social configurations in which they take place and make sense.

This relatively extended view on care pathways left one last question unanswered: what do the patients themselves say about what happens to them? With Solène Billaud and Pamela Skaff, I interviewed about twenty people, from the fall of 2015 to the spring of 2016, in the regions of Paris and Montreal. We discussed their past, what they experience, their daily lives, how they anticipate the future, and the people who help them. Most participants highlighted aspects of their history, even if they broke the thread of the conversation or repeated themselves to do so. Sometimes it was difficult to ascertain whether the participants were striving to put on their best faces or if they were suffering from relational difficulties associated with the disease. Ultimately, though, this was of little concern to us, as our sociological approach consisted in identifying and understanding systems of interaction, not judging what is normal or pathological.[7]

Investigating the Social Experience of Dementia: Theoretical Bases

The "experience of dementia" constitutes an area of interest in several disciplines such as psychology, social work, public health, and sociology[8]. Its exploration is generally based on interviews with patients and/or caregivers. The narratives obtained then tend to be analyzed in listing the main topics enunciated—for example, distinguishing between "it will get worse" and "I want to be me" and "nothing's right now," "I'm alright, I'll manage," "I still am somebody," and "it drives me mad."[9] The present research is complimentary to and different from these traditional approaches to "experience" because it combines multiple types of data collected in various places, and above all because rather than seeking to identity "phenomenological" topics, it seeks to describe processes occurring more relationally, within the "interaction orders." To be more specific, I will now present more clearly and formally this approach that I am developing.

(a) From the moment someone is suspected to suffer from dementia, the interactions they experience gradually change and a set of specific interactions gradually takes place around them.
With notable variations depending on their "culture" and social position,[10] concerned individuals are taken in a configuration that tends to repeat itself and thereby sediments in interaction patterns. This configuration engages both their possible interlocutors (whom the "patient" meets with) and the very form of the exchanges that occur with such interlocutors (including ways of communicating, expressing politeness, and making decisions). Often, family members start wondering what they need to do. They look for some information, eventually organizing themselves to provide care. They begin to act slightly differently. Professionals may also intervene. Leading such interventions are the doctors initially consulted for the diagnosis, closely followed by the employees of various health services who manage the consequences of the disease. This includes those involved in home care services as well as nursing homes and other aged-care institutions. Several devices shape this configuration. For example, local public policies, because they partly determine the framework of care, from "good practice recommendations" to health promotion campaigns, significantly shape the care configuration. Such devices all tend to define the set of values that orient the care process. They delimit a set of norms to be eventually followed and representations to be eventually appropriated.

(b) Individuals experience inseparably the progression of their disorders, called "symptoms," and the interactions they can live— the "interaction offer."[11]
In this typical "micro-politics of trouble,"[12] the "small things"— details that seem secondary at first glance, such as the manners of greeting, talking, smiling, or behaving—become prime objects of study. They are the very medium by which the illness stamps

its imprint on the social lives of patients. That is to say, there is no "cognitive loss" or "neurological dysfunction," such as memory troubles, that can be thought of as a pure, isolated, medical segment of reality, apart from the objects of these problems (what is forgotten?), their context (when, where, and with whom?), their management (set of behaviors provoked by the omission), and, eventually, anticipation—as well as all the social representations attributed to the actors, objects, and interactions at stake. Add to this the whole set of sometimes imperceptible changes in the patient's sense of self and self-presentation, reflected by the others, and the manifestations of these changes through intonations, words, hand gestures, and so forth. These "small things" thus grant us a perspective from which we can begin to understand how the social experience of dementia is produced: they partly *construct* this experience.[13]

(c) Dementia thus consists of a progressive shift, or distortion, of the interaction order.[14]

Therefore, *because* it investigates what Goffman calls the interaction order in the case of Alzheimer's disease, this book unfolds an ethnography of what Ian Hacking[15] calls the "looping effect": a systematic depiction of how categories interfere with an actual illness through everyday interactions. Note that despite the seemingly fanatical sociological dimension to this argument, it is congruent with a growing number of medical studies concluding the influence of the material and relational environment of the patient on the evolution of their disease. I hereby take some recent criticisms levelled within the sociology of health into consideration, according to which sociologists tend to be dismissive of the symptoms of the diseases they study[16] and omit studying how medicalization processes concretely impact the everyday lives of the concerned persons.[17]

(d) It is possible to retrace this shift in the interaction order through the multi-sited observation of various interactions experienced by (or taking place about) persons who are diagnosed with dementia.

Observing in multiple locations the interaction patterns unfolding around the diagnosed persons provides us with a vantage point from which we can explore the social experience of dementia. Thus the principal objective of this book is to propose an ethnographic account of what dementia *is*. This approach implies devoting greater space to immerse readers in the participants' narratives and observations, sometimes losing oneself in the stories of people who cannot completely fit with the slick analysis under progress. Delving into particular situations (which are not necessarily "representative") in detail will aim at highlighting a specific positioning: to be sure, sociologists are analysists of the social world but also and inextricably public writers of the present time, documenting contemporary social life. They are theorizing and describing in the same movement.

(e) The shift in the interaction order occurs through four recurring processes: the organization of repairing exchanges, the loss of credibility, changes in deferential behaviors, and reconstruction activities.

Following this method, the four chapters in this book account for four interactional processes that shape the experience of dementia. First, facing troubles gradually identified as symptoms, people see their daily lives threatened. A caregiving network—often composed of family members and/or professionals—is consequently organized, partly to remedy the domestic consequences of troubles. This is what I call the *organization of repairing exchanges*, and it is the primary focus of the first chapter. Second, professionals and relatives of the diagnosed persons tend to interpret some of their behaviors and words as manifestations of their illness. Patients thus suffer from a gradual loss of *credibility*. The issue of credibility and its contestation among the caregiving network is the subject of the second chapter. Third, the signs of *deference* developed toward patients change and become an issue. This is especially so in institutions, where the way in which staff members intend to protect the "dignity" of the persons is particularly pronounced. I turn to the topic of *deference* and its various instantiations in the caregiving network in the third chapter. Fourth, as the patients' ability to communicate diminishes, both their relatives and professionals attempt to maintain communicative exchanges with them. Maintaining communicative exchanges occurs through the partial *reconstitution* of what an interaction *would have been like* without the cognitive troubles the patient faces. That is, interactions are modeled on the forms of communication exchanged prior to the emergence of their troubles.

(f) In sum, considering that some interaction patterns repeat themselves around the diagnosed persons, and that this configuration necessarily modifies their (and their caregivers') relation to others, to themselves, and to their social world,[18] *we can infer from observations of this shift in the interaction order some knowledge about dementia as a specific collective experience of social life.*

FORGETTING
ITEMS

1

THE ORGANIZATION OF REPAIRING EXCHANGES

A RED FOLDER. IN A SMALL HOUSE ON the northern outskirts of Paris, a red folder sits on a round coffee table. The living room is perfectly tidy, almost unnervingly so. With the old furniture freshly dusted, an unmistakable odor of cleaning products lingers. On a shelf in the room, a few books sit meticulously ordered. On the walls, several family photographs pepper the dated wallpaper. An old clock announces the passing of time, *tick-tock, tick-tock, tick-tock.* As is the case with many newly diagnosed patients who have had to give up some of their activities and retreat to house maintenance, Mr. Chauffinier's house is impeccable. We sit around the round table, which is placed in the center of the room. Mr. Chauffinier keeps his prescriptions inside the red folder, along with medical examination results, lists of appointment with various doctors, and information brochures about his recently diagnosed dementia. Widowed for several years, Mr. Chauffinier is a former electrician and eighty-eight years old when we meet. Everything turns around the red folder. We don't know where to put our eyes during the discussion, and the red folder comes to occupy our gaze. Our interaction mediated by the red folder. For Mr. Chauffinier himself, the red folder and its precious contents provide the only informational horizon. Unfamiliar with the internet and anyone involved in the medical world, Mr. Chauffinier meticulously reads and rereads the contents of the folder, then carefully closes it and returns it to the table. After our conversation, it occurs to me that

Mr. Chauffinier perhaps sought some answers to his questions, some clarification of his troubles. When I turn off the Dictaphone, he hands me the folder. "I don't see how all this can heal me. I don't understand . . . What should I do?"

A folder is also present on the impeccable table of the equally impeccable living room of Madame Boisvert, a former teacher, who is eighty-three years old when we meet. She warmly welcomes me into her home in the suburbs of Montreal. We sit around the dining table to discuss. From time to time during the interview, her husband speaks a few words. Madame Boisvert opens and closes the folder that sits in front of us several times during the course of our discussion. A brochure from the Alzheimer Society, a Canadian community organization responsible for familiarizing patients and their families, catches her attention. She thumbs the pages anxiously. Giving an interview to a researcher is a potentially embarrassing affair. Interviews often involve speaking of one's difficulties and reflections on the past and the future—a future that, in the context of this particular interview, appears compromised. Having something at hand, something to read or feel while speaking, fictitiously disables this sense of embarrassment. Flicking through the brochure also makes broaching certain topics possible:

> [She stops speaking and starts to read. Silence for a few seconds]
> What stops me there is when I get to "health and personal care planning." That's what I say to myself, there, that's serious there. I'm not ready to do that, me.
> *Which is to say . . . ?*
> You know, when I'll no longer be . . . [pointing to a paragraph on financial guardianship]
> [Reading with her] *Able to take care of your bank accounts . . .*
> I've always done that by myself. . . . There's someone who'll make decisions for me? It doesn't interest me!
> *Yeah, I guess. . . .*
> I'm used to taking care of my own business! Christian [her husband], on his side, he does his business. Every now and then, I ask him for a little help, but I've got the last word about my business.
> [Silence, we read]
> "Health and personal care." Well, it means that maybe it's going to happen. Things won't always be . . . The momentum I still have, I still have a little bit of momentum. . . .

So what is it that is especially difficult? Is it difficult to imagine the future?

Yes, that's it . . . And then there's something else [reading the brochure]. What do they say? Like when I couldn't take care of my own affairs . . . "Financial and legal matters." I never liked those things! [She laughs]

Already, without any problem, it's boring!

Yes, that's it. Well, they say "financial and legal issues." I don't have much. I just have a bank account, that's all. . . .

Well, as you are married, it will be your husband . . .

Yes, he'll . . . [reads the brochure] "A power of attorney authorizing a person to make decisions on your behalf." I prefer it to be someone who lives in my house, or one of my children. I could trust each of my children. Oh yeah, that . . . They were well brought up! We didn't want them to steal from us when we got old! [Laughs]

But you have raised them well, so it won't happen! And you talked about that with your husband? The future and all that . . .

The future? No. I don't like that. I don't like to talk about that. But maybe sometimes, it would be better to take the lead. If I . . . what is . . . let's say, before a choice . . . I would like that.

For Madame Vanin, there is no longer any question of a folder. Her medical and administrative documents lie on the table in the living room, next to some photographs of the members of her family, carefully labeled so that she remembers their names and places in the kinship. Madame Vanin's home is also remarkably clean and tidy, maintained with the aid of a domestic helper who comes by several times a week. Medicines and medical equipment are stored on other furniture, mostly the coffee table, next to which a "comfort seat" (a voluminous wheelchair) sits. In the corner of the room, past the "comfort seat," lies a walking frame. In the background, a television program trails off, contrasting the still and silent atmosphere of Madame Vanin's home.

Mrs. Le Bordec describes how she has reorganized her home for her husband, since he experiences regular memory problems and finds himself disoriented quite frequently. She marked the corridors and the doors of her house with posters, indicating the rooms with the help of photographs. Same thing with the furniture: everything is now strictly tidied, drawer by drawer, with labels indicating what is inside each one.

The presence of medical documents, prescriptions, and information appear absent from Mrs. Fabre's home. She lives in a room in her house, where her son came to live with his wife and children in order to allow his mother to stay at home. Mrs. Fabre practices many artistic activities, and the room in which she lives contains many paintings, canvasses, and drawings—perhaps a curated selection of her lifework. Many photographs also decorate the walls, though unlike Madame Vanin, they have no labels and no names. There is nothing about any illness. Mrs. Fabre's son and daughter-in-law manage everything, probably in another room.

At Madame Corvisart's, who resides at home with the ongoing help of several professionals and her nephew (who is the only member of her family living nearby), there is no trace of medicalization. It is only after a meeting with the professionals working with Madame Corvisart that I realize that most of the prescriptions, boxes of medicine, and other medical documents are locked in a large plastic bag hidden on a top shelf so that the patient can neither see nor reach it.

In nursing homes, medical records and medicines are listed in alphabetical order and stored in offices that are inaccessible to residents.

From a folder placed on the living room table before a visit to an organization of medical objects across furniture, to the disappearance of these objects as they are managed elsewhere, the arrangement of interiors tells a lot about the patient's relationship to the disease and the organization of care. This first look at homes introduces the central focus of this chapter—namely, monitoring the steps that people diagnosed with dementia are going through, from the first symptoms to the diagnosis, from the first family reactions to institutionalization. This chapter shows how what I refer to as an *organization of repairing exchanges* establishes itself around each diagnosed individual. This organization aims to contain, as much as possible, the consequences of the disease on daily life, an organization that requires unequally distributed resources such as money, available relatives, and information[1] about health services.

The use of the term *repairing exchanges* seeks to reorient help and care practices in line with the main conceptual framework that guides this book, a framework grounded in the Goffmanian approach to interactions. More specifically, *repairing exchanges* are, in my vocabulary, a declination of what Goffman calls the "corrective process":

> When the participants in an undertaking or encounter fail to prevent the occurrence of an event that is expressively incompatible with the judgments of social worth that are being maintained, and when the event is of the kind that is difficult to overlook, the participants are likely to give it accredited status as an incident—to ratify it as a threat that deserves direct official attention—and to proceed to try to correct for its effects. At this point one or more participants find themselves in an established state of ritual disequilibrium or disgrace, and an attempt must be made to re-establish a satisfactory ritual state for them.[2]

This implies considering cognitive disorders associated with dementia as producing ruptures, transgressions, in the interaction order and activities aiming at correcting or repairing these transgressions.

Potential Patients

Who has never spent a few minutes looking for one's keys, glasses, phone, or credit card? Who has never struggled to remember a name or a face, finding oneself lost in a situation that one is supposed to know well? Most of these everyday scenes are not attributed any particular meaning, except when they involve a particular social group. This has led some entrepreneurs to invest in this "market of ordinary omissions," designing applications and devices that make finding one's keys, pets, and wallet much easier. For their part, psychologists have also suggested that among the working population, such temporary omissions and memory lapses could be a symptom of "burnout," or work-related stress. In their most acute form, such omissions and lapses constitute "legitimate" problems requiring consultation.

It is within this context that the Alzheimer's disease trajectory begins. The course has its origins in the "little things," in "little omissions," which tend to repeat themselves, occurring with greater frequency over shorter periods of time. "He did not know what day it was." "I could not cook anymore." "I forgot what I was just told." "We had to repeat the same things several times." Something, seemingly trivial at first sight, goes wrong. But future patients and the people around them, perhaps on account of the apparent insignificance of the lapses, rarely interpret these first troubles as "symptoms." They prefer other hypotheses, such as retirement, which can confuse people accustomed to work, stress, and transient depression. Other hypotheses proffered include the cognitive effects of diabetes, which can also provoke memory loss, or the death of a loved one, even a change of habits. In most cases, these troubles are initially normalized—that is, one may offer an explanation forged out of the pathological spectrum, but many hold that such troubles are not those associated with dementia.[3] This normalization can happen even when some uncertainties arise in the family, especially since a person can "hide the problems" for a long time in order to avoid a diagnosis.

The intense media coverage of Alzheimer's disease leads others into the office of a geriatrist at the slightest concern.[4] I once met a former high school teacher who complained fortnightly about forgetting where he put his keys. With the threat of early onset dementia, he rushed to his doctor only to be advised to consult a psychiatrist for anxiety.

How do we go from a series of ordinary troubles to a problem identified as falling within the remit of medical expertise? In other words, how does one *become a patient*? The initiative to see a doctor, mostly taken by relatives and not by the patients themselves, depends on two conditions: first, the observability of the troubles and second, the sensitivity of people around the future patient to the medical interpretation.

With the concept of *observability*,[5] I designate a *configuration* in which a trouble becomes potentially observable. This condition depends on the relation between the type of trouble and the domestic situation of the individual experiencing the trouble. Here, we can clearly distinguish between those who live alone and those who cohabitate with others, or at least those who receive regular visits. In the case of those who live alone, occasional memory losses may go unnoticed for years. In the case of those who cohabitate and/or receive regular visits, any problem, even minimal, can be spotted very quickly. Because some events reveal troubles and unusual behavior to relatives in a particularly striking way, observability in such contexts is drastically increased. This is often the case with family meals or trips:

> I would say that was, now, around three years ago. I took a holiday with her to France and Italy and I started to notice problems when we were packing and preparing. When she was choosing her clothes, she had some difficulties knowing how much to bring and I had to help her. . . . It's certain that, when you're with someone 24 hours a day, after a moment, there are normal conversation topics and after we made all of them, I realized she wasn't making a lot of the usual comments on what we saw. [Ms. Gosselin, physiotherapist, Quebec (research by N. Carpentier)]

Normand Carpentier's study of sixty family caregivers in Montreal shows that when the affected individual lives alone, the time elapsed between the first troubles identified by the caregiver and the eventual diagnosis is fifteen months on average. This is because relatives notice when domestic problems emerge and are more likely to send the affected individual to the doctor immediately. In contrast, the time between first troubles and diagnosis for those who live accompanied is on average twenty-six months. While relatives are more likely to identify the troubles earlier on, they worry less about the consequences because they are around to regulate and mitigate the possible damages. In fact, and this is a crucial point, troubles never function as autonomous problems. Rather, the troubles always fit in a configuration structuring the perceived degree of severity.

For example, the former chef at the Élysée Palace (the official residence of the president of France) wrote in his memoirs that Jacques Chirac liked to boil his milk by himself in the morning, but he would often forget it on the flame. Where this may have caused fires for "ordinary" people, a team of servants and assistants would, in Mr. Chirac's case, turn off the cooker.[6] Moreover, since the troublemaker was a busy man for socially legitimate reasons, everyone assumed that he had good reason to be "absentminded" in this way. A readily observable trouble but interpreted otherwise.

This aspect is precisely my second point. From the moment troubles are observable, and in order for the future patients to be successfully diagnosed, they or someone in their entourage will have to *interpret these troubles as requiring medical attention.* When the future patient already receives attention by one or more health professionals, observability and medical interpretation tend to be immediate. For example, physicians tend to very quickly assess residents experiencing memory problems in nursing homes. In contrast, the diagnostic process may take several months, even when the disorders are readily observable, in cases where future patients and the people around them produce and repeat nonmedical interpretations of the affected individual's troubles.

Furthermore, the interpretation process changes when a relative or acquaintance of the future patient is familiar with the symptoms of dementia and Alzheimer's, either through their own experiences or their awareness and understanding of the symptoms in other sufferers they know personally. The interpretation process is similarly affected in cases where relatives and acquaintances work in the medical world or related industries and environments (here, a good example is Mrs. Gosselin, previously cited, who "immediately recognizes" dementia-related troubles). In such cases, where the relative is associated with or otherwise involved in the medical world, not only is the medical interpretation facilitated but contacts and communication with specialized professionals can be accelerated. This is largely because the concerned people already know whom to contact.

> When he retired, and just before he retired, we had lived in the same semi-detached house on Doris Avenue for over thirty years. He walked past our door and went up to the second house, to the next door, and tried to get in. I saw him, I was standing by the garage and he didn't see me, and he tried to go in to that house. So, he missed the house and it's the only time he ever did in over thirty years. . . . I didn't know what else it could be, other than after he retired, right after he retired, he wouldn't do anything except sit and watch television. . . . I just got mad at him, because he had no interest and

all we wanted was freedom, he wanted his freedom, he didn't find freedom. Now, if I look back, I think that's probably a symptom. At that time, I thought 'ha, this is the classic retirement problem', particularly with men, no hobbies, no interest, all work, and suddenly they're cut and gone. . . .

What brought you to the memory clinic?

We heard of it before. I actually got Alzheimer information from the Alzheimer Society about a couple of years before because my mother-in-law was a candidate for it. Then . . . I guess when we started, when he started doing the car thing and missing the house . . . I, we maybe, we did suspect Alzheimer's and we didn't know that there was nothing we could do about it, but if we could catch something early, we might have a chance. So, and I knew the General Hospital had a Memory clinic, somebody told me about it. I've gone to social work myself a long time ago, saw the program at Dawson College and had some friends who worked in the General Hospital. So, we went to see Dr. Bern. [Mrs. Proulx, former housewife, Quebec (research by N. Carpentier)]

Lastly, because there is no remedy to date, as Mrs. Proulx notes, future patients and/or their relatives doubt the relevance of going to the doctor: what is the point of being alarmed if we cannot do anything about it?

The Diagnosis

While the increasing number of dementia diagnoses is certainly due to an aging population, there is also an important sense in which rising rates of diagnosis are attributable to other forces. There are two principal factors at issue here: first, the increase in diagnostic devices available to the medical profession and second, the interest of the pharmaceutical industries. With regard to the former, geriatricians in particular provide a specific medical context in which the issue of dementia finds a particularly acute form. In the latter case, medicine is not primarily prescribed on the grounds of effectiveness but rather to sustain or strengthen the relationship between patients and their doctors.[7]

The diagnostic process usually takes place in three stages. Initially, a patient goes to his or her family doctor, usually incited and/or accompanied by a family member. The patient or the relative speaks of the troubles he or she perceives or experiences. Sometimes doctors themselves initiate the diagnostic process, if on another occasion they have identified certain symptoms associated with a form of dementia. In any case, the doctor sends the patient to a specialized geriatrician or neurologist and prescribes the examinations required for these consultations (most of the time, a blood test and an MRI). Depending on the services, the patient might wait a few days or even up to several months.

Evry, September 14, 2011

Dear Colleague,

I am sending you, for a neurological assessment, M. Chauffinier, 88 years old, who complains of slight memory losses. MMSE = 25. What do you propose? The cardiac assessment is normal. The biological assessment is normal. There are no risk factors. I entrust him to you and thank you,

Best regards,
Doctor Manche.

The first "memory consultation" follows a specific protocol, which is more or less the same in Western countries.[8] The geriatrician or neurologist starts a conversation with the aim of obtaining some biographical information. He or she seeks information about the patient's domestic situation and cognitive state. He or she ensures that a sufficient set of aspects is covered, in order to develop a "global picture." As in the case of the consultation with M. Chauffinier, patients find themselves scrutinized on a number of themes, addressed point by point.

GERIATRICIAN: How long have you had memory problems?

PATIENT: Oh . . . for a year . . . one or two years . . .

G.: And it bothers you?

P.: Well, it's always annoying, memory . . .

G.: How did you realize that? Do you forget to post important mail?

P.: Oh no, when it's important, I do it!

G.: Do you forget to pay your bills?

P.: No, fortunately!

G.: Do you forget to turn off the gas when you cook?

P.: Oh no, otherwise I would set the fire to the house. . . .

G.: Do you forget people's names?

P.: Oh yes, that happens to me [he smiles at me].

G.: And your son realized your memory problems?

P.: Yes . . . but I also told him about it. . . .

G. And your friend?

P.: No, she did not say anything.

G.: Do you live with her?

P.: No, no, I live alone. . . .

G.: All right. And the kitchen, do you cook at home?

P.: Yes.

These discussions are interspersed with the reading of medical records and the examination of medical analysis results. Then a set of tests is performed, starting with some general tests such as the mini-mental state examination and the clock test. Depending on the situation and the outcomes of the general tests, the physician can then move to more specialized tests (TMT, verbal fluency test, Grober and Buschke, etc.). Finally, the physician synthesizes observations. The physician can propose a new appointment or new examinations, prescribe medications, announce a diagnosis, or offer some suggestions regarding the patient's homelife and organization. Usually two consultations are required for a diagnosis. Even when all the information is available from the first consultation, the doctor can wait for a second appointment to announce the final diagnosis. When there are no doubts from a medical perspective and the doctor considers it necessary, he or she can announce the diagnosis directly, especially in cases where there might be good reason to alert the patient or the relatives as soon as possible. As the label "Alzheimer's disease" tends to frighten people, doctors exercise discretion when informing their patients of their diagnosis, sometimes using euphemistic formulations for those who seem aware of their difficulties. This is what happens with Monsieur Chauffinier, whom the geriatrician finds reasonable enough.

GERIATRICIAN: Good. It is indeed memory that is lacking. Maybe [passing the tests] did not interest you, though? Still, it is the memory that poses the main problem. There are also some small language problems, and then difficulties with the clock [test], but that may be because you are left-handed. Did the test confuse you?

PATIENT: No, I was mistaken. . . .

G.: So it is actually a memory disease and a weakness of other functions. So I will prescribe some medicine that you will have to take every day. . . . [She tells him what to do, then comments] But you know, you're 80, if you would have had these difficulties at 60, it would have been much more serious, you know, age plays a role, but there, what you have, it's a little lower than . . .

P.: Than normal, yes.

Around this labelling process, a long and difficult period begins: progressively, in addition to managing everyday difficulties, the patients and their relatives have to reassess what to expect from their futures and redefine themselves within this newly qualified situation.[9]

A lot of practical problems arise unexpectedly. And each comes like a painful shock. Who will take care of the patient? Do we have the money to manage the potential costs implied by the disease? How long before the patient's state requires a 24/7 surveillance? How will the patient maintain a decent life? Can we keep our friends and our usual activities? The best way to illustrate this transition seems to present a particularly confused situation where none of these questions have been solved.

"Another Stage" after Diagnosis: The Example of the Levasseur Family

Mrs. Levasseur agreed to meet me after a conversation on the telephone. I obtained her contact details through the Alzheimer Society. She informed me that she would prefer that her husband be present for the interview. On a Wednesday morning, I made my way to a suburb on the southern outskirts of Montreal. The

Levasseur house is also the headquarters of the family construction company. I rang the doorbell. A woman greeted me at the door. She seemed stressed, even panicked. She appeared to be between fifty and sixty—too young for Alzheimer's, I said to myself. Was she the patient's daughter? Careful to avoid any blunders, I began to chat with her casually, and then, after five minutes, she invited me to sit at the table in the dining room "to do the interview." It was her.

I asked her to sign a consent form, but when I took it out of my bag, she panicked and exclaimed that she could not write anything. Finally she agreed to sign, managing—temporarily—to overcome her fear of "failing" her signature. Her husband arrived, greeted me, and went to another room. Mrs. Levasseur told me that we could wait to begin until he came in. I suggested it would be interesting to start the interview with just the two of us. She told me to wait for him. She went to get him, and they came back.

I found the house particularly well maintained. On the table, there was just a flowerpot and a folder. When Mr. Levasseur joined us, he opened the folder and took out a white sheet on which he noted my name. Throughout the interview, he went back and forth from the table in the living room to the kitchen, nervously leafing through the sheets he kept in front of him. The documents appeared to be some Alzheimer Society brochures and some pages printed from the internet. Mrs. Levasseur spluttered and sniffled intermittently. I did not know whether she had a cold or was constantly sobbing. Probably both.

Mrs. Levasseur had grown up in a small town of three thousand inhabitants in the Eastern Townships and eventually settled in the Montreal area in the 1960s. Born into a large family, she had been raised by one of her aunts, as her parents did not have the means to take care of her. She married in the early 1980s and worked in the family business. Until recently, Mr. Levasseur was in charge of the outdoor work while his wife managed the accounting and the secretary work. When Mrs. Levasseur worked in the family business, she often found herself supporting her husband's role—"I brought him the things he needed, the things that he forgot," she bitterly noted. The couple had two children; the first son became an engineer and worked in Montreal, and the second son worked as a police officer in another suburb. Each son had two children. The couple used to spend their free time doing activities organized by local associations: dancing, bowling, and knitting.

A few years earlier, Mrs. Levasseur had begun having trouble finding her words. Her sight had diminished as well. Moreover, she recounted some memory losses and orientation problems that disrupted her usual tasks. She said she no longer liked to cook—or, as her husband commented, "Was she less keen to do it, or was it because she had more difficulty doing it? Because when you have troubles doing something you are less likely to want to do it." Little by little, Mrs. Levasseur felt unable to pursue her professional activities. Keeping accounts seemed more and more complicated. As for leisure activities, she also found them gradually more difficult. Since she was relatively young when she initially noticed these changes (roughly fifty-five years old), diagnosis took a long time. Aside from a few ironic remarks from her grandchildren ("that's it, you've got Alzheimer's!"), no one imagined that she could really be suffering from a form of dementia. She went through numerous exams—several kinds of medical imaging and then a lumbar puncture—before the family doctor concluded a hypothesis of dementia and sent her to a memory clinic.

The diagnosis came on March 14, 2015. "We were not expecting that," said Mrs. Levasseur. Depressed, she cancelled her driver's license: "I never touched the car again. It was finished. Driving was causing me too much stress. . . . Because I had problems with my eyes, I got honked at regularly, you know. So I said, look, it's enough."

In the course of our conversation, Mr. and Mrs. Levasseur insisted on their attachment to certain leisure activities, discussing how the activities helped them to make friends. Mr. Levasseur recounted that in order to continue practicing some of his hobbies, he had to let some other ones go—which is a common experience for many caregivers.[10]

> I think there are still some great moments to live. It's just an adaptation there. . . . So I do some activities. I gave up some others, because I did a lot, a lot. And I dropped a lot . . . because . . . on Monday, I

go bowling, on Monday afternoon, so I come back at 4:00 p.m. On Tuesday . . . I have some dance, so I leave at 9:30 a.m. and I come back at noon. That, I let go. I said to myself, "It's okay, I'll let it go." I told myself, on Thursday afternoon, dance, I will let go of that too. I still have . . . on Wednesday morning . . . I go bowling . . . so I have Friday, Saturday, and Sunday when I'll be here at home, and on Tuesday I'll be here, then Thursday . . . but . . . we'll still see a show on Friday, a show on Saturday, a show on Sunday . . . and just before we go to do some shopping. I said to myself, we'll go check out some sweaters. . . .

This reorganization of activities is certainly quantitative (what you do and do not do anymore), and this excerpt suggests Mr. Levasseur put a lot of thought into these decisions; they are also qualitative in the sense that it means something different to each member of the couple, now that time and energy are seriously limited resources, to pursue or not to pursue an activity. It probably involves more of their self-feeling, the proof that there are still "great moments to live," and the notion that they can still have "time for themselves." While Mrs. Levasseur gave up dancing because she could no longer dance easily, she dropped her other activities because she feared rejection and the difficulty associated with regular attendance. She found it difficult to follow the activities, feeling unsure about her capacity to participate. In particular, a negative experience with her knitting comrades made her fear that a similar situation could reoccur. She was told that her husband had "contaminated" her. (This is the only time I heard this belief that Alzheimer's disease was contagious.)

Mr. Levasseur decided to stop working in the winter of 2015–2016, a less active period in the construction industry, in order to stay with his wife. I met the Levasseurs in January 2016, and they were unsure of how they would fare when summer returned. This apprehension was particularly acute because Mrs. Levasseur could no longer bear staying home alone, and the disease led them to question their source of income.

> Mr. Levasseur: I have no idea what she could do . . . no idea what she could do. . . . She was doing crossword puzzles, but she doesn't anymore. . . . It's hard. . . . Word search, she doesn't do that anymore, it's difficult. . . . She does her best, she does her best.

Because you, as you work in construction, have to go to construction sites, I suppose?

Yeah, exactly. I will leave at 5:30 in the morning and come back at seven in the evening. There, I don't know. That's why I wanted my guy [son] to take over the company, and I would be a company employee, that way I'd have more time. But we're not there yet. It takes time, but I like that I would have less to do.

Do you think taking over the company would interest your son?

Yes. He will attend some classes. Though at the same time, he could have something else in mind, because in the winter, [business] is hard. . . . There's work, but there is not much in winter. It's hard to do, it's hard to do. If there is anything else to do during the winter, it could be in home automation or something else. . . . You know, he could add this business.

So he may modernize the company as he takes it over.

Yeah, that's it, and me, I could help him for three or four years. . . . It would give me more time.

Was it planned, that he'd take over the company? Or did you accelerate it because . . . [undertone: of the disease of your wife]

No, he talked to me about it a year ago, then I thought he wanted to take it quickly, but there were unforeseen events. Toddlers, you know. . . . If he doesn't want to take it over, I will not sell it. . . . It's here, it's my name.

Mr. and Mrs. Levasseur had occasional contact with a few health professionals, mainly the family physician, the neurologist from the memory clinic, and a researcher conducting a clinical trial. Their children and grandchildren visited them regularly. Additionally, they received some support from the local Alzheimer Society. One of the employees of the local Alzheimer Society came to see Mrs. Levasseur from time to time ("we talk about how I feel . . . and if . . . what I plan to do"). Mr. Levasseur also took some educational courses that he drew on extensively during the course of our interview. This intense assiduity gave me the impression that the medical discourse, in proposing a legitimate, dominant model of diseases, may offer people some meaning to hang on to in difficult times.[11]

[She passes a] lumbar puncture to see how she evacuated depending on the proteins in her brain. All that . . . because in your brain you have proteins, so your cells can function, but they do not circulate well, and depending on that they can know if you have [inaudible] or not. And [inaudible] it means that the proteins there will cluster around your neurons, your synapses, all that stuff, and in the long run it will make plaques. And the plaques are going to prevent the cells from working. And, more than just working, to succeed . . . to live. So they're going to die. They will die in groups, depending on where your brain is being attacked. And, well, every place in your brain has a human function. It can be walking, it can be understanding, memory; in a corner it can be mathematics; it can be anything. Even if you were very good at something, normally when you were very good at something you might be keeping it longer, but it does not mean anything. This something can diminish anyway.

For a couple accustomed to leaving the house regularly and attending a certain (gendered) distribution of activities, Mrs. Levasseur's troubles gave rise to a redefinition of daily life and professional routine, which was still under discussion when I met them. In light of the changing configurations of daily and professional life, Mr. and Mrs. Levasseur called a housekeeping service to solve the household problem, though they quickly cancelled it because the employee did not seem "professional" to them. They therefore found themselves in a situation in which they had to discuss and rediscuss the terms of their common life repeatedly. It is probably for this reason that the interview regularly slid into settling accounts. The couple oscillated between expressing their fears, accusing each other, and formulating their ongoing domestic issues.

Mrs. L.: Well, you would have liked it better if it fell back [if the disease would have affected the back of the brain]. I could still be able to calculate—

Mr. L.: Hell no! I would have liked it better if you had nothing at all! Don't say that I would have preferred you to lose memory or I do not know. . . . The less you lose the better it is. [To me] that's sure. It's been three, four years since she last cooked a meal . . .

[. . .]

Mr. L.: No, me, it didn't bother me. I thought that since she had done so much cooking [in our conjugal life], it was really appropriate that I do it, even if during the summer, as I work, it's harder for me.

[...]

MRS. L.: Well, regarding food, they say that if I forget something it might start a fire, so, that . . . You know, those things could happen. Marie [the Alzheimer's Society employee], she says it's better that I do—

MR. L.: No, but this is in the immediate future. Otherwise, three years ago, let's say, we couldn't understand each other. I said, "Look, I stop working in the winter." I stopped working in the winter, and I did the food. She was happy, and it's okay. Then now, well, the summer arrives and we'll . . . I do not know.

[...]

MR. L: Then, since she does not cook anymore, so, me, I try to do what she—

MRS. L.: Me too, I would like to do—

MR. L.: No, no, but it's okay, I try to do.

MRS L.: What do you want . . . I don't mind washing the dishes . . .

[...]

MR. L.: We don't know where we're going, but we'll see. That's why I'm taking courses, to inform myself, to be able to tell when we're at another stage, and look, you might need someone who comes to help you with the housework. Home care.

MRS. L.: I am still autonomous.

MR. L.: Yes, but now we are just talking about it. We're just talking.

The early years during which patients and their families try to adapt to a new, ever changing situation is also a period of anticipation: what could happen? Characteristic of this stage is the upheaval of daily and professional lives, brought on by the diagnosis and symptoms of a family member or relative. The story of Mr. and Mrs. Levasseur, which is somewhat atypical since Mrs. Levasseur is fifty-seven (and only between 1 percent and 2 percent of diagnoses occur before age sixty), reveals how uncertain the domestic reorganization process is, what feelings and logics it engages. In this transition period, repairing exchanges fundamentally are attempts. As a consequence, this configuration structurally produces blunders and embarrassment. The way in which Mr. Levasseur repeatedly summarizes their situation seems an appropriate way to negatively define this troubled time: "We are in another stage."

The Development of Caregiving Networks

Diagnosed individuals experience a *loss of autonomy*, a term used mostly in public health discourses. Experiencing a loss of autonomy means that it is no longer possible for patients to live alone in their own homes and that respecting certain standards of safety, hygiene, and comfort become increasingly difficult. They have to resort to the help of others, in much the same way that children or persons with severe disabilities are often required to have carers and assistants. These "care" or "assistance" roles entail the labors of domestic monitoring and basic living support. This can be a challenging and difficult situation to accept for patients, largely because this change occurs in a broader social context in which autonomy is celebrated as a value. "We" consider that individuals must be autonomous, manage themselves, think, and be responsible for their situations. In its most concentrated form, this is the ideology of the *self-made man*, the man who made himself and who needs nothing from others.

Such idealization of autonomy frequently overshadows the fact that other social groups regularly make use of different carers and assistants to maintain their lifestyles. Well-to-do families may use domestic workers, and it is not uncommon for middle class families to hire house cleaners or gardeners. Celebrities require large entourages and surround themselves with multiple coaches. Government's highest officials receive luxury assistance services, such as special hairdressing and cooking. Medical services and support networks are regularly rolled out for presidents and ministers. Furthermore, mutual support schemes often appear in couples or families—for example, couples might have their child cared for by their parents, or a partner (women in majority) may help to prepare for his or her loved one's upcoming workday, for instance ironing shirts and making lunch. In fact, while our societies erect autonomy as a value, the number of people who rely upon autonomy as a practice is relatively low.

In order to situate people diagnosed with Alzheimer's disease in this general system of dependencies and assistance, we must distinguish between two types of assistance. The first type of assistance *defines* the persons who receive it; for example, "children," adults "with a disability," the elderly "in loss of autonomy." The second type of assistance does not influence the definition or prestige of those who receive it, although it is often necessary to maintain their position (adults using services). Furthermore, the discretion of this second type of assistance seems to be a condition of its social efficiency. For example, some servants working for the haute bourgeoisie report how they have to do their jobs while being invisible.[12]

Most people diagnosed with dementia occupy a particular position in the mode of production of wealth. They do not work while they receive help, which places them in a situation where they cannot justify the help received by an imperative of production (but such a distinction remains porous, if one thinks of the aristocracy).

Given this, how do domestic changes take place around patients who are losing their autonomy? As their ability to perform day-to-day activities is compromised, family members who reside with them or within close proximity generally have to take on more tasks. In couples, where the distribution of domestic activities is strongly gendered, these changes sometimes involve interesting reorganizations—men who have never cooked begin to cook, women mow the lawn for the first time, and so on. When the diagnosed person can no longer drive or faces driving prohibitions, the relatives' intervention tends to intensify, especially when shops and services are far away. When relatives cannot provide assistance for whatever reason, patients can resort to of professional services. However, such services are not within financial reach for all patients. If patients cannot afford professional assistance and if, as a result, they miss important information regarding financial support opportunities—as in many contexts the organization of health services is experienced as a "maze"[13]—their living conditions can rapidly deteriorate.

The interview with the Levasseurs illustrates that in addition to domestic tasks (housework, cooking, dishes, etc.), an intense reorganization of recreational occupations may occur. Mr. and Mrs. Levasseur sacrificed certain activities in order to preserve others. Similar processes of reorganization and sacrifice affected Mr. and Mrs. Le Bordec, who presented their daily life as largely centered on travelling. The Bordecs had to reduce the frequency of their trips and the distance of their destinations, from the whole world to Western Europe. For aged people whose lifestyle is more sedentary, this process consists of the reorganization of leisure activities. For example, an individual might stop reading and devote more time to watching television. This process can also concern professional life—for example, in patients who are still active (they must resign, if they are not fired) or for the family caregivers (typically, the spouses move to part-time employment or leave their jobs).

Improvements to the patient's domestic configuration can also facilitate aid. For example, labels affixed to objects, enabling easier identification; installing support bars and handles throughout the home when cognitive disorders are coupled with proprioceptive issues; or even alarm systems that indicate potential hazards. In the case of alarm systems, relatives and professionals often associate a patient's reluctance to have them installed with a form of "denial," but this attribution ignores the extent to which the implementation of such devices affects the patient's social image:

[In the office of a geriatrician, January 2012]

DOCTOR: Mrs. Benaji, it would be nice to set an alarm in your house. Just in case—

Ms. BENAJI: No. No. It is a matter of self-love here. I don't want that in the town. They take me for a dum-dum.

All these changes to the patient's domestic configuration involve a modification of the care network constituted by relatives and professionals as well as the relationships between them. Initially, some relatives get involved by providing small services, such as bringing a meal from time to time or going to visit the diagnosed person, which intensifies in follow-up visits. Other relatives withdraw and quit completely, like the nephew of Mr. Le Bordec, who emailed to explain that he had to "take some distance" because they no longer had "the same way of life".

In our society, the members of the nuclear family (couple + children) are generally considered responsible for acting in the first place. This responsibility is coupled with a second norm concerning territory, which is to say the closer one lives to the diagnosed person, the greater the expectation that they will help. Moreover, a third standard involves the material resources of the potential caregivers, which includes professional status, economic situation, and health. The support of professionals, whether doctors, home-help services, or local associations, depends on the structures available in a given territory and their accessibility. In other words, the form of support is contingent upon the information possessed by the care network, the price of the services, and the information on financial assistance for those who cannot afford such services.

While some care networks seem to organize themselves "spontaneously"—as is the case when each member of the network assigns themselves given tasks—other care networks formally organize themselves, either through meetings or a schedule system. When the resulting configuration is problematic for some of its members or observers (for example, the neighborhood), professionals can take over the organization of the network. This is largely the function of the case managers. Case managers are co-ordination specialists established in most Western countries under various names and institutional conditions.

Despite being able only to summarize the main parameters involved in the help configuration, it is nonetheless possible to observe some recurring dynamics. In very simple terms, I will first distinguish two crucial roles that are present in each case. First, "whistle-blowers" are those individuals, typically family or close friends, who regularly evaluate the patient's condition and whose presence in the affected individual's life often catalyzes the diagnosis process. Moreover, whistle-blowers often alert other potential caregivers of the changes required in the patient's care. Second, there are "decision-makers" who—as the name suggests—are those who make decisions. These two roles can be occupied by different persons or simultaneously by the same person:

(a) In some "centralized" configurations, only one caregiver is both a whistle-blower and a decision-maker. This generally occurs when a widowed patient has a single child living nearby or when the patient's spouse is in good health. This is the case for the Levasseurs and the Le Bordecs, where the spouse, despite receiving occasional help from the children, takes full responsibility for the diagnosed person. By definition, few conflicts occur, but the caregiver has a good chance of "cracking" at a certain point.

(b) In configurations where several people are both whistle-blowers and decision-makers, a sort of "oligarchy" of caregivers sets up. For example, this occurs when the diagnosed person lives alone and several children organize themselves together to try to deal with the situation in an egalitarian way. Since it is rare for everyone to agree on the required help, this type of configuration tends to turn into a "decentralized" configuration (see the next section). Ms. Bonnefont recounts how her brothers and sisters mobilized at a certain point:

> Actually, each of us, we saw there were some problems with our mother. We organized a family meeting, with my brothers and sisters, to share all our experiences. We said: "How do you find mom?" . . . Everybody didn't see the same things, but from the moment when we met up, it started. It's like we realized that she needed help and that it wasn't about exchanging anymore. I mean, in the past, with me, because I lived nearby her home, we used to help each other. [Research by N. Carpentier]

(c) Finally, there are "decentralized" configurations where several people are whistle-blowers and decision-makers, but they rarely hold both positions simultaneously. For example, this configuration can emerge when the person receiving the help has several children, one of whom lives closer or considers herself or himself to be the favored child. In these cases, there is only one whistle-blower (the closer child) and several decision-makers (all the children). This creates some discrepancies, as Mrs. Côté told us:

> They went to see the geriatrician in Maisonneuve. They made him pass some tests, the famous sheet, that exam [probably referring to the mini-mental state examination]. Following this, he [the geriatrician] met my brother and my sister who were with her [the patient],

and he told them, "Enjoy the good time you have with your mother, because she is at stage four." They came back home and they called us all, but I was not surprised because I expected that. I had been telling them for the past three years that there was a problem. [Research by N. Carpentier]

This analysis of the dynamics of power in help networks enables us to clarify two types of conflicts that frequently arise. First, there are conflicts linked to a disagreement among decision-makers and whistle-blowers, who compete for the fate of their relative, which is most common in "oligarchic" networks. Second, there are conflicts regarding the extent of the help configuration (for example, when the whistle blowers do not succeed in mobilizing as many caregivers as they want), which are more likely in "centralized" or "decentralized" networks.

The most in-depth studies on the topic (considering both francophone and anglophone literature), that of Florence Weber, Agnès Gramain, and Séverine Gojard on family care and that of Aude Béliard, which deals specifically with Alzheimer's disease,[14] show that conflicts arising within help networks generally stem from social cleavages and differences in the family. Indeed, when one family member becomes dependent on the others for assistance, old quarrels and disagreements may reemerge. In certain circumstances, resurfacing disagreements may reinforce the exclusion of a family member who has experienced some social mobility. In other cases, confronting old disagreements can retrench preexisting internal (social) divisions within the family.

Trouble Management and Material Configurations

By what "features" does the domestic organization of the diagnosed persons evolve? What social conditions shape the support they seek[15] and can have access to? The comparison of two situations will provide the way toward an answer.

I met Mrs. Vanin during a visit from her case manager, who had been working with her regularly for over a year. Despite their regular contact over the year, Mrs. Vanin did not, at first, recognize her case manager. Mrs. Vanin was a former secretary and lived in a house that she had built in 1964, situated on the periphery of Paris near a small town with around ten thousand residents. She had moved to the area because her in-laws resided there. Prior to his death is 1985, Mrs. Vanin lived with her husband, who worked as a mechanic. Born in 1929, Mrs. Vanin received regular visits from a housekeeper who came to clean and run errands as well as visits from a nurse, a physiotherapist, and her family doctor, who delivered her medications.

Mrs. Vanin's situation had changed a year prior our interview. She found herself hospitalized for several months following a fall. During her stay at the hospital, she was diagnosed with dementia, as her cognitive troubles became suddenly observable and interpretable in the hospital configuration. After her stint in the hospital, she went home. However, she did so without knowing how she could possibly live there. Mrs. Vanin could no longer walk, and her big house was situated on sloping ground. To access the front door, one had to climb two stairs, which were not accessible with a wheelchair. Moreover, Mrs. Vanin required assistance to get up every morning. When she came back from the hospital, she gave her car to her neighbors. Her granddaughter, Nathalie, took care of her for some time but could not maintain support as she resided 150 kilometers away and also had to take care of her mother (Mrs. Vanin's only daughter), who suffered from multiple sclerosis and lived in a specialized facility. Mrs. Vanin's only sister and brother-in-law, with whom she had strong ties, died prior to her diagnosis. One neighbor provided some occasional help, bringing cooked meals from time to time. But all in all, this was not enough support to enable her to stay at home under conditions that would be considered decent.

Mrs. Vanin also tended to give money to all the salesmen who knocked at her door and generally tipped fifty euros to the paramedics who took her to the hospital for her appointments. She regularly forgot who was who. Her grandchildren were worried, and the manager of the home help sector in her area contacted a case manager, who tried to recruit a home helper for several hours a day. However, local social services were overwhelmed. Mrs.

Vanin's case manager then sought to ascertain support from social services that would assist her in avoiding being placed in a nursing home—an outcome that everyone around her was striving to avoid. Her grandson, who visited her once every fifteen days, had been assigned guardianship in order to prevent her from giving too much money to strangers.

During the interview, it was obvious that Mrs. Vanin was terribly bored. She could no longer leave her home and enjoy the activities she loved:

CASE MANAGER: And now, what do you do during the day?

MRS. VANIN: Well, you know, not much. Not much.

CM: Sure. The day is long.

MRS V.: Yes, yes. I try.

[Pointing at a TV magazine on the table] You watch TV?

MRS V.: Yes, but actually I'm not connected. I don't look at it all day. A bit in the morning or at lunchtime, yes, sometimes more in the afternoon, depends on what there is.

You were involved in more activities before? More leisure activities before?

MRS. V.: Well, before I worked outside a lot.

Ah, the garden?

MRS. V.: I was maintaining it. I didn't do everything but still. I mowed the lawns; I did a lot of things. Now, all this, it's over. . . . On the whole, I'm ok anyway. But sometimes I put myself on the edge [of the window], just to see the moment simply, to see what happens.

During our conversation, she expressed mixed feelings about the care she received. She felt alone but did not dare to call her grandchildren and neighbors. She was worried about calling them too often and was concerned not to disturb them, not to be "a burden." Like many people encountered during the course of this study, she advanced a form of modesty: "You know, I'm content with little," she said. "I get used to everything." On a few occasions, Mrs. Vanin noted that she would like to have fewer professionals around her while explaining that she had no choice but to stay at home. She said that what disturbed her most was being placed under guardianship: "Judicial representatives and all that, I don't like being too much . . . I like to be free to do what I want. What I want . . . ah . . . what I can." "It's very embarrassing. . . . You have to understand me. . . . You have to understand me." She noted that, even if she had to stay in her home under guardianship, her priority was to avoid ending up in a retirement home. "I will go on like this until the end."

Madame Fabre's case was very different. Eighty years old when we first met, Madame Fabre had spent most of her life in Paris, in an apartment. She had worked for many years as a nursemaid in the welfare service, which meant that she welcomed children in her home for long periods (several months or years). One of her employer's requirements was that she regularly take the children to a country home. Madame Fabre was granted credit to buy a house with her second husband, who worked as a teacher and passed away after they acquired the house. Madame Fabre's father-in-law sold them the land "at a reasonable price." With her second husband, she spent weekends in the countryside and, when retired, settled at the house full-time. Madame Fabre has five children from two marriages: one son lives in Guadeloupe; another son is institutionalized in a center for "mental retardation"; one daughter lives in Paris; and the other lives in the Parisian suburbs. Her youngest son moved into her house, with his wife and two children, some years ago in order to provide the care that she required and to prevent Madame Fabre from being institutionalized.

As a result, her son and daughter-in-law handled most domestic tasks, along with the occasional help of their sixteen-year-old son. In addition to the help provided by family, Madame Fabre went to a day hospital twice a week. According to her case manager, her attending the day hospital gave the family some respite. According to Madame Fabre, she believed herself to hold a different status than the others: "they [the staff members] take me as an assistant"; "I make the elderly sing . . . as my mother sang in cafes." She regularly received help from a housekeeper from the town hall as well as home nursing services. Accustomed all her life to practicing various artistic activities, she did not lack leisure activities. She painted, did embroidery or collages, and drew, sometimes with her grandchildren. But I did not know whether the paintings she showed me were recent. Anyway, her room was full of these works.

Mrs. Fabre affirmed that she contributed to family life, for example by helping with cooking. She added that even if she went to the doctor for testing, she would have "passed well." Mrs. Fabre's case manager told me that she had been diagnosed with a form of dementia and that she was, in fact, not able to cook and now posed other problems. Mrs. Fabre had mood swings and sometimes insulted her daughter-in-law. Consequently, her relatives found the situation difficult to manage and began reluctantly planning a nursing home placement in the coming months. Still, at the time of our interviews, Mrs. Fabre appeared unperturbed by these issues, or at least did not speak of her perturbation. During the interview, she avoided topics relating to the disease or domestic difficulties and focused instead on her present or past occupations: "Yes, I do small things. I do painting, I do painting, I knit, and I collect the little cats that are abandoned. Well, yes, because people are moving! And then the cat is not always there when the car leaves."

Let us compare the situations of Mrs. Vanin and Mrs. Fabre. For the most part, professionals surrounded Mrs. Vanin while Mrs. Fabre enjoyed continuous family presence. Mrs. Vanin was affected by both mobility problems and memory problems while Mrs. Fabre moved well. However, Mrs. Fabre's cognitive difficulties had recently been coupled with aggressive behaviors. The domestic configurations and the resources of each patient differentially shaped the relation between their troubles and their help networks. For example, the two women owned houses, but owning a house presented a handicap for Mrs. Vanin (her stairs preventing her from going out) while for Mrs. Fabre owning a house was beneficial, allowing her to live with her family. Mrs. Fabre's home was comparatively much more modest, located on the ground floor and without stairs. The women's cultural affiliations also differed. Mrs. Fabre's prior artistic activity enabled her, in addition to keeping herself occupied, to keep face during the interview and to present herself in a favorable light while Mrs. Vanin expressed, above all, her feeling of boredom. In both cases, they were taken care of and no longer made decisions about their lives.

As the illness progresses, patients tend to find themselves "stuck" in their homes, and so their relationships to spaces are crucial components of their stories. Their lived territories, the ones they actually frequent, tend to diminish as their cognitive states worsen. Recall Mrs. Levasseur, who attended several activity groups in her town and visited local shops by car. When the effects of Alzheimer's reach an advanced stage, lived places are no longer cities or urban spaces but rooms or, indeed, only parts of rooms. For Mrs. Vanin, as for many people "stuck" at home, the lived places consist of the living room, the bedroom, the bathroom, and the edge of the window, where she can observe the trees, the weather, the people, and cars passing by.

Simultaneously, a patient's attachment to the home is reinforced because the home takes on a different meaning. Many of the people interviewed boasted about the quality of their houses or apartments, repeating how well maintained they were. Typically, some said they still took care of the housework when I ask them what they did, and then later they explained that they employed housekeepers to do it. Demonstrating that one still knows how to "hold one's house" is essential, especially for women socialized into the expectation that they are principally responsible for maintaining the home, even more so when the home is a family property.

More importantly, to emphasize how pleasant one's home is conveys a certain message. That is, repeating that one is "at home," that one is "lacking nothing," that one is "satisfied with little," and that one "doesn't complain" even when the situation proves difficult amounts to a refusal to be placed an institution.

This explains why housing can be a sensitive issue. Mrs. Corvisart, a former bank employee in her nineties, seemed completely disoriented when I met her. She forgot the people around her every five minutes, including her nephew, and hardly answered my questions. Yet she reacted very sharply when I asked her a simple

question regarding the domestic configuration, as if she were suddenly too upset to have symptoms:

> *Do you like your home?*
> [Frowning, talking louder] Where do you want me to go?
> *Well, I don't know—*
> Not in a nursing home, I hope?
> *No . . . I hope not. . . .*
> I hope you don't think about that!
> *No, I don't think about that. . . .*
> [Firmly] Because I'm well here.

Placed in Institutions

While the number of nursing homes is certainly increasing, the ex-
clusionary processes that render some individuals "outside" of traditionally understood domestic orders are not a new phenomenon.[16]
However, the leitmotif of the discourse surrounding contemporary
nursing homes no longer centers on the explicit exclusion of these
people from the society they disturb (which they always do, in fact)
but rather affirms the development of more comfortable, more secure
forms of everyday life, preferable to the living conditions at home. It
is within this context that we can observe the relatively recent development of specialized units in nursing homes. These units are devoted to residents diagnosed with dementia or those suffering from any
cognitive trouble. The introduction of these specialized units accompanies a wider array of services and facilities specifically targeting
those individuals diagnosed with dementia and similar cognitive disorders. Such services and facilities include specialized architectural
forms, such as buildings organized in a circle that permit residents to
wander in a harmless setting. Various security devices inspired by the
prison and psychiatric worlds, such as electronic bracelets and self-
closing doors, are also used. Furthermore, this new configuration
also encompasses the development of specific activities and reserved
places, such as cognitive stimulation workshops, "Snoezelen spaces,"
and "reminiscence spaces" (rooms decorated to evoke the past).

A minority of people decide to get placed in nursing homes.
Of those who do, the principal motivation is to attenuate their feeling of loneliness. The majority of those placed in nursing homes,

though, are there reluctantly or even against their will. In all cases, the possibility of being placed in a nursing home appears to patients, their family, and the health professionals around them as a last resort. Many end up in nursing homes; once placed, they become *residents*. In this new context, the organization of repairing exchanges, which has so far operated through multiple trials and errors, becomes institutionalized. It now follows an upstream, planned organization of work.

Residents experience the arrival in a nursing home as a biographical turning point. Indeed, it is a break in their social trajectory. Prior to entering the nursing home, their social status was associated with their income, their assets, their profession, and their marital status. Although this status affects the selection of which institution they are placed in and the progression of their health, from the moment they enter a nursing home, the opportunities for them to evolve in this social microcosm are extremely limited. What limited form of social mobility there is in the nursing home consists of "moving" into a unit reserved for people in a state considered worse than their own.[17]

In a given ward, all residents receive similar treatment, in more or less the same way, by the same professionals, in the same infrastructure. Contrary to life outside the walls, differences in treatment within an institution depend, in principle, on the state of the patient's health, not on their social position. Residents keep only a few items from their previous lives—some clothing and decorative objects for their rooms. Residents also receive money, akin to the way teenagers receive pocket money, to be used to purchase additional food, items, and services.

Statistical research shows that institutionalization is linked to age, domestic difficulties, and the severity of the patient's symptoms.[18] If we examine these factors closely, we can identify four types of evolution leading to the institutional placement. In the first scenario, intensification of symptoms produces a burden perceived as too heavy for the caregivers. Here, caregivers "crack" after spending enormous amounts of time and energy maintaining their relative's lifestyle at home. Such "cracks" often occur when problems of incontinence, hygiene, and sleep escalate. In the second scenario, reduction in professional interventions makes the consequences of the disease unmanageable for the members of the family. In the third scenario, a change in the caregivers' lives (for example, death, sickness, or a new job) can make ongoing care for their relative increasingly demanding and thus unsustainable. In the fourth scenario, the person receiving help faces hospitalization for physical or mental health problems, after which the option of returning home is ruled out. This can occur because the hospitalization accompanies a clear increase in the disorder or because hospital staff members convince the family that a medical environment is necessary.

In each of these scenarios, there is a "straw that breaks the camel's back," so to speak, which is often the result of a long process in which caregivers have entertained the possibility of institutionalization for several months. Since institutionalization is expensive and often requires family members to make significant financial sacrifices, caregivers proceed in the decision-making process in several stages. The work of Solène Billaud deals with issues of financing placement in France in more detail.[19] Billaud brings to light the "symbolic economy of 'small goods'" which occurs upon the patients' institutionalization. Relatives share what belonged to the institutionalized person as a "semi-inheritance"; the furniture is allocated by a random draw and the objects allocated according to the affective and utilitarian values they hold for each member of the family. Billaud shows that at this point, because they are under the gaze, albeit distant, of the person being institutionalized, family members try more than usual to "make a family." That is, to stage their good relationships, even when conflicts divide them the rest of the time.

In this last stage of the dementia trajectory, the help network remains mobilized around the resident, but often with less intensity. The staff members of the nursing home replace the role of home professionals, although some home professionals may continue to visit the resident from time to time. All the modalities concerning the residents (medical records, medicines, administrative papers, etc.)

are centralized, now being managed by the employees of the institution, with the possible participation of relatives. Activities available to the patient are planned, organized by the staff, and "adapted" to the disorders. However, residents tend to devote a growing part of their days either to wandering in the corridors, waiting in a chair, or sitting in front of a television or a window.

Conclusion

This chapter proposed a broad outline of the organization of repairing exchanges established around persons initially suspected to be suffering from dementia and then eventually diagnosed. Such organization aims at "limiting the damage," at "repairing" disturbances to daily life, and sometimes at anticipating the troubles in the interaction order. It creates patterns of care that permeate the experience of the illness—notably as they structure what form, effect, meaning, and consequences symptoms *can* have in social life. Furthermore, this set of material possibilities and representations is grandly limited by the "context," social and historical.

Regarding the historical aspect, we shall mostly consider that we are facing a particular generation—namely, those people born in the years 1920–1940, who share social experiences characterized, for the most part, by long periods of full employment and relative stability in terms of access to work and housing (which could constitute an additional explanation for their special attachment to their home).[20] This generation also shares the experience of transitioning into "old age" at a specific historic period. More specifically, they transition to "old age" at a time when Alzheimer's disease has emerged as a public health issue and when specialized devices for tracking and managing the troubles associated with the disease are developing. This is indeed the first generation for whom dementia represents a large-scale mediatized threat. Therefore, this generation is simultaneously more "informed" than the previous one and less "prepared" than the following one because the associated services and support infrastructure is still in the process of being established. In sum, this generation enters "old age" during a time of transition, between the growing recognition of age-related cognitive disorders by medicine and public authorities (1980s–1990s) and the building of large-scale institutions and devices aimed toward managing dementia as a public health issue.

Recognizing the contours of this historical situation sheds light on the case studies presented so far. In a context of fear and unpreparedness, it is unsurprising that the help provided to diagnosed people occurs with multiple hesitations. These hesitations can be identified in the reluctance to define the "nature" of the disorders and in the often-conflicting negotiations about the daily life to which the diagnosed person can aspire to, and regarding the possible and doable help configurations.

As these hesitations subside, as the troubles develop and the caregiving network gets organized, especially around risk management, the patients have less and less say—I do not mean that they have no agency in itself but that the conditions for such agency to exist socially decrease.[21] Of course, money helps some to pay for professional help, which diminishes the domestic consequences of troubles and the burden borne by family members. But it does not help resolving some ethical problems then arising without any solution over the horizon. When patients express their wishes, such as a wish to avoid being placed under guardianship or a desire to remain at home despite increased risk of accident, people around them tend to consider that this decision is not their own, "for their own good."[22] Ultimately, what takes precedence is the assessment by others of the patient's requisite care. Because at a certain stage, conceding the slightest margin of "freedom" amounts to enabling injury or even death.

2

LOSING CREDIBILITY

FROM THE MOMENT A PERSON IS SUSPECTED TO be suffering from dementia, the interactions they encounter begin to change. And among the changes that occur, one of the most significant is *the loss of credibility.*

By credibility, I mean the fact of being believed by one's interlocutors. When the people you talk to consider your words and gestures valid information, or at least "authentic" manifestations of your "personality," this means you are credible. Most interactions operate on the basis of the implicit assumption that people are credible,[1] which interlocutors tend to stage through gestures such as nods, attentive glances, or any other sign that emphasizes that they are taking account of what is stated.

Nevertheless, this postulate may be called into question every now and then, typically when lies are disclosed or, more consistently, when a whole person's character is questioned. Thus, certain highly ritualized exchanges consist of explicit tests of someone's credibility. This happens in the cases of criminal prosecutions (does the accused tell the truth?), appointments with social services (do the users describe their situation adequately?), job interviews (do the prospective employees have the skills they claim?), and psychiatric and geriatric consultations (is this patient "crazy"?). Each of these rituals operates according to precise institutionalized standards regarding what makes someone credible or what discredits them. For instance, in the immediate court appearances observed by Lara Mahi,[2] individuals cannot prove that they are ill by showing the judge physical signs of their illness. Rather, they must provide official documents that substantiate a medical diagnosis.

Some populations have their credibility systematically called into question. This is often the case for psychiatric patients, individuals whose spouses are particularly jealous, and elderly people suspected of suffering from dementia. In the case of those suspected of suffering from dementia, people around them tend to assume that this or that behavior says less about a "genuine" facet of their "identity" and more about the behavioral manifestation of some cerebral malfunctioning, a raw display of the disease. During my research, many family caregivers and professionals spoke of their reluctance in having their loved ones or patients participate: "He will tell you anything." "She's no longer able to realize what's going on."

In certain situations, such as trade negotiations or electoral campaigns, it is well known that protagonists arrange their presentations of facts for particular strategic ends. We are culturally equipped to recognize these situations, to decode them and tolerate them to some extent. But beyond that, when someone is suspected of not being credible for a long time, that they have been discredited deeply changes the relationships they can experience. All the relationships of this individual become problematized through this prism.

Such discreditation relies primarily on language. When a person is supposed to be credible, their interlocutors tend to interpret what they say and do as descriptive acts, which they can integrate into what they know about this person. In these cases, the function attributed to language is the same for all: to describe a reality, to give it a meaning. However, when a person's credibility is in question, the content of their discourse is understood as the manifestation of something else. For example, the content of a discredited individual's discourse might be pinned down to a pejorative trait (for example, dishonest merchants who lie about the products they sell) or a disease. In our case, people diagnosed with dementia talk about their daily lives and their desires, but their interlocutors often consider these words signs of their trouble rather than pure expressions of interiority. Language itself becomes a symptom.

The discovery of a lie can color a whole relationship and can reverberate far beyond the moment in which the lie is unveiled. In the same way, although people around patients do not attribute to patients responsibility for their disorder, discrediting their expressions and behaviors nevertheless radically transforms these relationships. The patients' interlocutors forget, little by little, that the patient can be credible. In such circumstances, interactions function without the usual assumption of credibility. The dementia trajectory can therefore be understood as a long process of discreditation, a nonlinear series of interactions in which people around the diagnosed individuals believe them, disprove them, ignore them, pretend to believe them, do not pay attention to what they say anymore, and so forth.

What Is Discredit?

If the first interactions with a specialized physician are a turning point in the trajectory of those affected, it is not only because they face the threat of being diagnosed with a disease that compromises their future. It is also because this meeting may constitute an initiatory experience of what it means to interact while being discredited— what is more, by a very legitimate professional, often in from of a significant relative who is sometimes discredited as well.[3]

The probability of being discredited originates in the diagnostic process itself. From the medical perspective, dementia has the particularity of not being detectable by means of obvious biological markers. For example, in Alzheimer's disease, only an autopsy can establish diagnostic certainty. Physicians must therefore manipulate several types of information and correlate them in order to produce an ultimately probabilistic diagnosis. This set of information includes the discourse of the patient and their relatives, MRI, blood tests, neuropsychological tests, and, more rarely, lumbar punctures. In this context, the construction of a clinical picture requires gathering the words of the patient and their relatives. These are the only means of accessing the difficulties experienced by the patients in their daily lives, as these difficulties do not always correspond with what the results of MRI or neuropsychological tests reveal.

However, a particular difficulty is that if patients actually suffer from cognitive impairment, it may mean that some of what they say does not reflect their "real" situation. Consider a case where a patient claims to have no difficulty managing their life at home when in fact they are encountering numerous difficulties. Believing the patient's words could potentially have dangerous consequences. In addition, one of the symptoms of dementia is "anosognosia." This medical term denotes a neurological dysfunction manifested by the negation of or refusal to acknowledge one's difficulties. If a patient denies having cognitive troubles, physicians may consider this denial a symptom. Hence, there are many reasons that lead health professionals to perceive the entire behavior of patients as a possible sign of illness. In this sense, then, *giving credit or discrediting patients is a condition of medical work.*

How does the passage from credibility to discredit occur? In the observed consultations, patients were encouraged to have close relatives accompany them. When a patient comes alone, the doctor "suggests" to them, with great insistence, that they return accompanied. In fact, the accompanying person is very useful to the physician in that they can confirm or deny what the patient says. Thus, the structure of the conversations between physicians and patients illuminates how patients see their credibility suspected:

[Fictive example based on observations]

DOCTOR (TO PATIENT): Do you cook at home?

PATIENT: Oh yes! I love cooking!

DOCTOR (TO THE ACCOMPANYING PERSON): No problem on this side?

ACCOMPANYING PERSON: No, it's okay.

In another case, patients find their role diminished as the accompanying person becomes the principal source of information. Patients are thus rendered almost useless:

[Fictive example based on observations]

DOCTOR (TO THE ACCOMPANYING PERSON): She cooks when she is at home?

ACCOMPANYING PERSON: Yes.

PATIENT: Oh yes! I love cooking!

Sometimes patients do not need relatives to contradict them. The inconsistency of their own words makes doctors discredit them. This often happens when patients speak of performing certain tasks and then say the opposite or undermine what they have spoken of at a later point in the conversation. For example, one patient explains that she does all her grocery shopping herself and yet, only five minutes later, complains that she cannot carry a bag. In another example, a patient recounts that she takes care of her large garden but later claims that she has difficulty bending over.

Finally, certain behaviors are associated with symptoms of dementia, especially when they corroborate other types of evaluations (neuropsychological tests and MRI). For physicians, these behaviors can be signs that the patient is not credible. Short-term memory loss, which is typical of Alzheimer's disease, is the best known example of a kind of indicative behavior. Moreover, short-term memory loss can be quite concerning if the results of medical imaging tests display subcortical atrophy. The forgetting of rituals such as birthdays or other ceremonies constitutes a symptom common to all types of dementia. In patients with MRI results indicating vascular lesions, "overly colloquial" behavior and poor results in verbal fluency tests are taken to be symptomatic of vascular dementia.

For over a century now, anthropologists have worked tirelessly to demonstrate that medical judgments amplify certain cultural expectations. While among indigenous Australians transgressing social norms, such as pronouncing the name of a deceased relative, may be one of the symptoms of age-related "madness,"[4] in Western societies other expectations prevail. For example, *coherence* in the presentation of the self is not only expected, but its failure is considered potentially pathologically abnormal. This expectation for coherence appears clearly in many social spheres. Carolina Kobelinsky shows, for example, that asylum seekers are partly assessed according to the perceived adequacy of their testimonies and attitudes. The employees of the French National Court of the Right to Asylum take into consideration displayed emotions (showing sadness when telling a sad story) and also physical appearance ("frankly, this one didn't look gay," an employee comments about an applicant claiming to be a victim of homophobia[5]). The medical consultation reproduces the same type of configuration. The difference, however, is that the doctor's judgment is based on tools that quantify, or stage in a technical way, the degree of the patient's compliance with cognitive norms.

Once discredited, the rules of interaction change for patients. These changes can occur suddenly, as I have observed with doctors during consultations, or they can occur gradually, as is often the case with family members, who try to adapt their behavior to the evolving condition of their relative in a piecemeal fashion.

One of the first changes to occur in a patient's new interaction order is when interlocutors begin to vary the intonation of their voice, or adopt a more contrived speaking voice. This type of intonation is referred to as *secondary baby talk*. Interlocutors may also increase the volume of their voice, even in cases when the patient does not have hearing problems. The ostentatious use of onomatopoeia and gestural communication reinforces this language, as well as the use of the third person singular to designate somebody in their presence, either in the indefinite ("are we doing well today?") or defined ("how is she today?") form. However, in our case, this attitude goes hand in hand with the assumption that the affected person does not hear or understand the discussions. In addition to these changes, frequent repetition of the person's name, closer physical proximity to the patient during conversations, and accentuated expressions of the face (in particular smiles) also occur with greater frequency during conversation.

Changed expectations shape the interpretation of the content of the patient's verbal expressions. As is the case with children, those in dialogue with discredited individuals tend to consider their activities "playfully," as if they are never truly serious, or as small quirks to deal with, and that the disease alters the judgment of the discredited individual.

Finally, the behavioral changes described here are also evident (but maybe to a lesser extent) in regard to the undiagnosed elderly. It is as if these behaviors all draw on the same "behavioral repository." This consistency across interactions with elderly people suggests that interactions experienced by diagnosed and undiagnosed older people tend to become more uniform with aging.

A Normal Life: The Example of Mr. Dupond

Each case of discreditation involves several recurrent features: how the visibility of symptoms is managed, what their effects imply in the domestic organization, the diagnosis itself, the convergence between what is said by the patient and what is reported by relatives, the patient's social position, and so forth. But the way in which all these features intertwine throughout individual histories is unique. Discredit can successively (or at the same time) be enacted, resisted, embraced, rejected, and laughed about or trigger tears. When Mr. and Mrs. Dupond enter the consultation room, they probably do not expect to play such a wide panel of emotions and situations revolving around the discredit of the husband. Narrating their consultation offers a compelling case of the social drama characterizing the discreditation process.

Mr. Dupond is a man of small stature, bald, and sporting a very thin moustache and round glasses. He wears a brown sweater and trousers of the same color. In his left hand, he carries a large plastic bag containing piles of medical records. Mrs. Dupond wears a scarf, a brown sweater, a watch, and some rings. Throughout the interview, she keeps her hands clenched on her purse that rests her knees.

The couple immediately unpack the plastic bag and place their medical documents on the doctor's desk. The paperwork piles high, about ten centimeters. Mr. Dupond splits the documents into heaps. On the upper half of the first pile sit the results of X-rays and MRIs. Mr. Dupond reaches for the large envelope sitting atop the stack and hands it to the geriatrician. The doctor thanks him and examines the pictures in the envelope.

We wait a few minutes. Mr. Dupond, who smiled and threw me some playful glances when he entered, comments, "We still have a small piece of brain, don't we?" While Mr. Dupond appears determined to relax the atmosphere, his wife does not seem to be in the same mood. Perhaps she does not like his humor. It is impossible to know. Anxiety distorts her face, she has nervous ticks, and her lips are constantly twitching. I do not understand whether she approves or disapproves of her husband's attitude. While Mr. Dupond positions himself slightly askew, elbow on the desk as if he were at the counter of a bar, she remains strictly straight and frozen, still with concentration for the entirety of the forty-five-minute consultation. The second stack of medical records contains envelopes of smaller sizes: prescriptions, doctors' letters, blood test results, and other papers. The geriatrician takes some time, about three minutes, to read the most recent results and letters. Meanwhile, Mr. Dupond appears uncertain and shrugs a little. "I don't understand anything," he seems to express as he spreads and stretches out his palms while shrugging and looking at me. He smiles at me, and I smile back. From time to time Mrs. Dupond, with her eyes fixed on the medical records and jumping at every "mmm, yes" of the geriatrician (who seems to read worrying information), turns her head and gives a disapproving look at her husband, who appears to oscillate between laughter and anxiety.

"Well," the geriatrician says, resting the files on the table, "tell me why you are here."

Mr. Dupond, still smiling, replies, "Well, I am here because I have memory loss. I do a lot of things, but I have memory loss."

The geriatrician frowns, I assume because the patient seems unconvinced by what he has just said. "When you came here a year ago, what were you told?" The geriatrician phrases the question relatively cautiously. Indeed, while the geriatrician reads that Mr. Dupond's medical record indicates a previous diagnosis of "beginning mixed dementia," she also knows that the patient previously consulted one of her colleagues and that doctors do not always give the exact diagnosis. She considers it best to address the patient directly, asking him what he knows and trying her best to avoid any blunder.

Mr. Dupond answers, "Uh, I was shocked to hear her saying 'early Alzheimer's.' But what really bores me is the loss of memory. . . . Otherwise, I have a normal life. Totally normal . . . " Silence.

In a serious tone, the geriatrician says, "You understand, Mr. Dupond, that this disease now accompanies you . . . all your life."

The man pushes his hands out again, palms upward, underscoring his incomprehension. "Yes, but . . . [resignation] I want to believe you doctors, but I have a normal life . . . "

His wife begins to tremble with emotion. She exclaims, "No, he doesn't accept it! He doesn't accept it!" She begins to cry. "He doesn't accept it. When we talk about it . . . he always redirects the conversation."

Mr. Dupond stops smiling and speaks more slowly. "Yes, I accept. I'm not a doctor, but I have a life . . . " Mrs. Dupond puts her hands on her face in an attempt to mask her distress.

"Well, I just looked at the medicines you take. . . . Okay. . . . Antidepressants? You've had depression," says the geriatrician.

Mrs. Dupond whispers between two sobs, "Yes, there were moments, moments where we went off the deep end." Mr. Dupond offers a mumbled "yes" and then stays silent. The geriatrician questions them about the effectiveness of the treatment. Mr. Dupond seems convinced of its effectiveness. Mrs. Dupond, however, is much less convinced. The geriatrician addresses her: "the disease also affects the center of emotions. It's mainly the memory that is affected, but the brain is a very complex organ. Everything is intertwined. It can reach the center of emotions too."

Tension now occupies the room. Mrs. Dupond cracks and bursts into tears. I think it would be indecent to continue taking notes, so I rest my pen inside my notebook and place it in my lap. I wonder whether she feels what has been sometimes observed in the literature: that spouses experience the disease as a sort of grieving process in several steps.[6]

"Sir, you know that with medicine . . . medicine preserves you for a while, but it cannot regenerate what is lost," the geriatrician says gravely. Mr. Dupond, apparently jaded, reacts with a wave of his hands and sighs. I still cannot grasp the emotions expressed by

Mrs. Dupond, who asks about advice previously given by a speech therapist. She wonders whether she should heed the therapist's advice and not correct her husband when he drives the wrong way. The therapist informed her that this would enhance his independence. The geriatrician asks for an example. Mrs. Dupond replies by referring to "an historic domestic fight" about driving. The patient addresses me: "Even if you are young, you've probably experienced this, no?" I laugh nervously. He then turns to his wife and says, "Yes, you see, he knows that too, even if he is young." Then, in a tone suddenly very serious, he says to the geriatrician, "Listen. I've been driving for several years . . . many decades! And never a single accident, not even one. I am careful, and especially that, yes, there is my wife, I am not alone . . . and I could stop. If one day I see that I can't, I will stop, but now I can drive. . . . Wait, I've been driving for forty years and not a single one—"

"Fifty years," Mrs. Dupond interrupts.

She is, in turn, interrupted by the geriatrician: "So, if it comes from you, so much the better. But this is not always the case." The geriatrician informs the Duponds about a service that tests the elderly to determine if they are still able to drive.

Mr. Dupond responds, "But I take no risk. If one day there's a problem, I'll see it!"

Quietly, the geriatrician continues, "Mr. Dupond, one of the characteristics of the disease is that one cannot evaluate risks. It's not your fault. It's the disease; it's not you. It's not your fault, but you may nonetheless be unable to assess your difficulties—"

Mrs. Dupond interjects, "But I think we need each other." Mr. Dupond smiles and holds out his hand to his wife. Affectionately they take each other's hands. "We've been together so long, so . . . Yes, we work together, that's for sure, we are . . . [gesture expressing a link]."

The geriatrician proceeds, "Well, do you mind doing some tests, to see where you are in terms of memory?" She asks Mrs. Dupond to leave the room. Mr. Dupond hastens to comment, "She's a bit rough sometimes. . . . My wife tends not to realize that I have troubles doing certain things."

"Realizing and accepting are two different things, Mr. Dupond," the geriatrician replies firmly. The man leans back in his chair, muttering something, and then calmly answers the doctor's test questions. He gets suitable scores, achieving 27/30 on the mini-mental state examination (results under 25 are deemed worrying). The geriatrician offers to make an appointment with the neuropsychologist at the hospital in order to get Mr. Dupond to sit for further tests that are "more at his level."

"Okay," he responds. "But I'm glad I did the test. It allowed me to spend twenty minutes alone in the presence of a beautiful woman.'" He laughs.

The geriatrician exclaims "Alone? [Pointing to me] There is the young man too, eh!"

Mr. Dupond replies, "Yes, but without my wife. You know, I like to joke. It's not mean. If my wife had been there, it wouldn't have been the same. [He smiles at me and winks] You know it's just that I like to joke."

The geriatrician responds coldly, "Well, I will go to inform your wife about the caregiver support program. I really think it will do her some good." She leaves the room to fetch Mrs. Dupond.

With the geriatrician now out of the room, Mr. Dupond, without provocation, launches into a real monologue. First, he tells me about his professional career, which was marked by social upward mobility. He started "at the bottom of the ladder," helping on construction sites, and ended up as a technician. Finally, he talks about his local reputation. He has lived in the same city for a very long time and has been the longtime coach of the local soccer club. Everybody, he says, calls him "Béberre,"[7] but his wife does not like this nickname. He complains about his wife. He likes to joke, he says, but his wife thinks that it brings them shame—which, gauging by the success of Mr. Dupond's attempt at a joke with the geriatrician, seems a likely outcome. He asks me if it is wrong to make jokes. Unprepared for his question, I hastily answer in the negative.

The geriatrician comes back with Mrs. Dupond, who just agreed to join the caregiver support program. The patient is looking for humor. "Uh, so I'll be alone for an hour a week. I can watch football games!" His wife gestures for him to stop, but she laughs a little at the same time. The doctor begins to renew Mr. Dupond's prescription. Meanwhile, Mrs. Dupond asks whether it is appropriate to double the sessions with the speech therapist, as proposed by their general practitioner, especially since "it has been going well."

Mr. Dupond exclaims, "Oh, I'd like to go there twice as much. I won't say no!" Intrigued, the geriatrician asks him why. "Well, I have to say that she's a very beautiful woman, eh!" He starts laughing. He winks at me.

Mrs. Dupond, to the geriatrician: "Yes, I have to admit . . . " Then, turning to her husband, a little annoyed: "But the important thing is that going to the speech therapist allows you to get better."

The patient does not miss this opportunity to joke again: "Well, I feel better now." Mrs. Dupond shoots him a dark look.

From then on, Mr. Dupond never ceases joking. He seems intent on doing so for my supposed benefit, since he jokes to the geriatrician and then laughs, looking at me for validation. Visibly annoyed, the geriatrician rushes to finish the prescription, concluding the consultation by insisting that Mrs. Dupond attend the support program.

After the consultation, I talk with the geriatrician. She explains how, in the waiting room, Mrs. Dupond confided to her that the couple have lost all their friends. They had walked away when Mr. Dupond started "losing his head." She expressed her anger: "they're all jerks," she said. The geriatrician and I share our impressions about this "exhausted" woman, who seems "close to the tipping point." According to the geriatrician, the patient is "disinhibited." In neurological terms, this means that he suffers from deficiencies in the brain system responsible for inhibition (in other words, self-control), which is characterized by greater ease and less discomfort in social interactions. This corresponds with the numerous vascular lesions visible on the MRI. These lesions are characteristic of vascular or mixed dementia. I relay to her what the patient told me when she was with his wife, suggesting that perhaps he had always liked to make "subtle" jokes. She concludes, "Okay, but I don't know him, and have you seen how familiar he was with me? No, no, that's for sure: it's vascular."

The Latch Effect in the Discreditation Process

Once discredited, patients face enormous difficulty having their credibility reestablished. This characteristic seems self-evident in the case of dementia, as symptoms are, for the most part, "incurable." Without the possibility of "getting better," patients are continually held to be unreliable. This "latching" effect is also observable in other contexts involving discrediting labels that are difficult to remove, such as psychiatric institutions or criminal justice systems. From a medical perspective, "anosognosia" consists specifically of the patient's denial of difficulties. As a result, not only does no one seem to believe that Mr. Dupond is leading a "normal life," but the more he claims it, the less credible he becomes. This inverse relation is also observable when Mr. Dupond attempts to prove that he remains a sociable personality in his town because his friends call him "Béberre" and that such joking remains a competitive endeavor among his friendship group. And yet, the physician associates these behaviors with the vascular lesions visible in the results of the MRI, which consequently solidify her discreditation of the patient.

Within configurations of discreditation, interactions raise serious questions of interpretation. In observing geriatric consultations, I noticed that the vast majority of patients frequently attempted to disrupt the course of the conversation set by the physician. Patients sought to talk about certain aspects of their lives, tell anecdotes, make some jokes, and so on. Physicians, who admittedly found these digressive attempts amusing at times, had to reframe the conversation several times in order to obtain information more directly relevant in clinical terms. In previous work, I have labeled these deviations "lost talks."[8] I opt for "lost" because they mostly pass for uninteresting ramblings and are, moreover, regularly lost in the thread of conversation. But what if we take these digressions seriously on terms separate from the clinical context? What is interesting about these discourses is that they are interpretable, schematically, in two ways: as the ramblings of elderly people losing their minds or as what remains of their "identity." More precisely, there are of four kinds of digression.

First, there are *childhood memories*, which consist of taking an expression out of its context and redirecting the conversation toward the evocation of these memories. While she passed the verbal fluency test with her geriatrician, Mrs. Berry used her score (13) to start a conversation. Mrs. Berry reflected on the day of her birth: "Thirteen . . . It's because I was born on Friday the thirteenth! It was a day when my mother . . . " Her son, who accompanied her to the consultation, sighed loudly, interrupting her. The geriatrician ignored the digression and asked the son to recount some anecdotes attesting to his mother's memory loss. From then, Mrs. Berry remained silent until the doctor directly requested she talk. This type of situation is profound: while patients are largely evaluated through the prism of their short-term memory, attempts to remind others that they can relate distant events may be a way to symbolically reverse the direction of the discussion and their diagnosis.

Second, and similar to childhood memories, there is *evidence of good conduct*, which consists of taking an expression out of its context and redirecting the conversation to show one's qualities, for instance a healthy lifestyle. During his first consultation with a geriatrician, for example, Mr. Duchesne did not succeed in articulating the three words he had to remember a few minutes earlier for a test. His face changed abruptly. After a few seconds of silence, the doctor gave him a clue: "There was a vegetable, for example. Remember the name of the vegetable?" Another pause. Mr. Duchesne was visibly embarrassed: "There, it is a black hole." The atmosphere becomes heavy. The geriatrician coldly replied, "It was . . . spinach." The patient exclaimed, "Spinach, yes! Spinach, yet I eat some, eh! I eat vegetables, and often spinach. Oh yes, but . . . a vegetable, spinach, and yet I eat!" The doctor interrupted him and asked him if he could remember the other two words.

Third, there are *shows of force*, which consist of imposing a manifestation of skill during an interaction. I identified very few examples of this type. However, the most emblematic belongs to Mr. Muller, a ninety-year-old former professional boxer who constantly sought to recall this aspect of his life. He stood slightly leaning on his side, his arm resting on the back of the chair. With exaggerated sympathy, I wrote in my notebook, "Al Pacino in *Scarface* but with fifty years more." This attitude also attracted the sympathy of the accompanying nurses, who are usually silent and reverential. This time, however, the nurses joked abundantly with the patient. Several times during the consultation, Mr. Muller proposed to "put on my shorts" (his boxing trunks). At a certain point in the discussion, his son, who was present, reminded him that he was "no longer able to get into the ring." Annoyed, the nonagenarian muttered, "You'll see if I'm not able!" He then got up, linked his hands behind his head, and bent until his elbows almost reached his feet while keeping his legs straight, as if to display his flexibility and prowess in the ring. He repeated this gesture several times with a display of flexibility that no one in the room would have suspected. Surprised, we all remained silent for several seconds, in awe of the elderly man's nimbleness.

Last, *showing detachment* denotes moments where patients indicate that they do not attribute importance to the questions addressed to them. Thus, patients try to demonstrate that they can rise "above" or "beyond" what is happening in the consultation. Detachment is understood here in the sense of what Goffman[9] calls "disengagement." However, the detachment illustrated does not necessarily indicate the patient's inability to remain focused during interactions (a possibility Goffman highlights) but can potentially be considered a deliberate course of action. Some patients show themselves openly disillusioned in front of everyone. Mrs. Bonvoisin, for example, deliberately amused herself. When her geriatrician began to give her a test, she answered, "You know, I have my temper, because . . . what? What's the question? Oh, you know, your test there, I don't give a shit . . . [To me] And you there, how old are you?"

Childhood memories, evidence of good behaviors, shows of force, and detachment are interpretable as attempts to gain credibility or at least attention. In their deployment, each form emphasizes more positive aspects of the patient's identity compared to those highlighted by medical evaluation. Yet these attempts are doomed to fail. As in the case of Mr. Dupond, they in fact end up consolidating the doctor's suspicion that the patients clearly have a problem, precisely *because* they are supposedly rambling. Even when the patients' behavior arouses some admiration, as in the case of Mr. Muller's gymnastics demonstration, such displays nevertheless strengthen the diagnostic apparatus of the medical professional. Though significant, admiration is not straightforwardly conducive to increasing one's credibility.

Unequal Facing Discreditation

During consultations, the social milieu, national origin, and gender of patients influence the relationships with the physician and affect the susceptibility to being discredited. First, in the case of a patient's social milieu, people with lower levels of education are more systematically discredited than others—a phenomenon that is also confirmed by quantitative research.[10] Geriatricians are aware of this problem and try to adapt the diagnostic process to the "cultural level" of their patients. However, Aude Béliard[11] has shown how the act of assessing the "socio-cultural level" produces an inequality regarding the certainty of the diagnosis reached. In other words, the assessment of a patient's "socio-cultural level" affects the diagnostic outcome. Béliard has also demonstrated that the way in which the elderly word their troubles (in terms of "memory" or "madness," etc.) varies depending on their social position.

In my observations, I have witnessed how the patient's socioeconomic level influences the course of the consultation *and* the opportunities that they have for maintaining their credibility. Yet such effects are apparent only when the elderly are in very high or very low socioeconomic positions.

In the case of "low" sociocultural positions, patients suffer from discreditation because the consultation poses particular challenges on account of their relatively poor command of language, both written and spoken. After having received Mr. Raulin, a former construction worker who left school at the age of ten, a geriatrician told me that she was skeptical about the real value of the test results: "with this kind of patient . . . it's true that there's an inequality because . . . this gentleman, he hardly knew how to read the tests. . . . When he said he reads [a newspaper], I would first wonder whether he can even read."

Ms. Najda, who lived a large part of her life in Algeria, speaks minimal French. She has never been to school and never worked. For her, passing the mini-mental state examination is a significant challenge. Her daughter has to translate the examination into Arabic at times, and Ms. Najda seems not to understand the purpose of such a test. In response to some questions, she answers "Insha'Allah" several times. Some tasks are impossible for her to put into practice (such as writing a sentence) or require important changes from the initial test. One task consists of showing the patient a poster with the phrase "close your eyes" printed in large font. In this case, the doctor is simply telling the patient to close her eyes. Presented with this poster, Ms. Najda responds initially with, "But I do not know." During the mental math test, which begins with the question "what is one hundred minus seven?" Ms. Najda's daughter tries to help her mother by placing her in a practical situation: "You have a hundred euros and spend seven. How many remain?" Facing her mother's hesitation, Ms. Najda's daughter perseveres: "You see a hundred euros, the green bill, and you take away a small bill and a big coin. How much do you have?" The doctor murmurs, "I can't believe that . . . " Ms. Najda continues to struggle to answer. From that moment on, she faces complete discreditation. The geriatrician now addresses only her daughter, interrupts the tests, and seeks the service of a neuropsychologist who speaks Arabic.

Most of the time, working-class patients "betray" their sociocultural origin in a much more anecdotal way, and geriatricians try to adapt. Mr. Alberti, a former mechanic, is asked to remember the word *armoire* during an examination:

DOCTOR: So . . . there was a piece of furniture . . .

PATIENT: Oh yes! A closet!

D.: Uh . . . not exactly . . .

P.: Well I don't see then . . .

D.: It was *armoire*. It's almost the same. What do I put?

P.: Oh yeah! Armoire, it sounds . . . better . . .

D. [LAUGHS]: Yes, it's . . . more chic, say! Come on, I won't count it! [She gives a point.]

In regard to patients that present in a visibly "cultivated" manner, their specific concerns often lead doctors to assume a pathological anxiety. Mrs. Phan, a former teacher, suffers from memory troubles. More specifically, when she reads novels in several volumes, she no longer remembers the names of the characters of the first volume when she passes to the second and third. She receives a referral to visit a psychologist. Another situation suggests that "excessive" cultural capital may also contribute to discreditation. For instance, sixty-one-year-old Mr. Dampierre complains of significant memory loss that is endangering people around him. Moreover, Mr. Dampierre's memory loss instigates constant reproach from his wife, whom he is divorcing at the time. Yet the doctors do not recognize these disorders. Mr. Dampierre passes his tests without any difficulty, responds faster than I could, and obtains excellent scores. In consultation, he is very agitated and offers multiple concrete examples to show the truth of these memory losses, despite the results of the tests. The doctor thinks that these problems stem from his divorce and that he should see a psychologist. Later on, when I meet Mr. Dampierre at his home to conduct an interview, he provides me with some explanation as to why medical professionals are disinclined to diagnose his troubles. In addition to graduating with numerous qualifications (business school and photography and graphic design studies), he had an impressive career in one of the biggest French companies before becoming its chief import-export director. He tells me that when he started to take up important positions, in a context of fierce competition between executives, he had to pass tests that were much longer and more complex than those conducted for the assessment of memory. "Four-hour tests, with three hundred questions," he said. In other words, Mr. Dampierre indicates that he is overtrained to pass tests. We may assume that such training impedes the medical recognition of his difficulties. Moreover, Mr. Dampierre's protracted reflections on his problems give the impression of a deep anxiety, which leads medical professionals to propose psychological intervention.

The cultural capital of the patients thus plays an important role in the possibility of maintaining credibility or, more precisely, in the different ways of losing it. Possessing a very "small" amount of capital, as in the case of Mr. Raulin or Ms. Najda, is systematically discrediting. Signs of "too much" capital, as with Mrs. Phan and especially Mr. Dampierre, can be interpreted as manifestations of psychological issues. Contrary to what is generally observed in medical sociology,[12] I argue that in this case, it is not the social proximity with doctors that plays in favor of patients but their "cultural goodwill," which Bourdieu identifies as "characteristic" of the lower middle classes.[13] Reacting consensually to medical expectations and abstaining from "rambling" seem to be part of the minimum requirements in order to maintain credibility in memory consultations.

Importantly, gender also influences the outcome of these consultations. It is worth noting, though, that the methodology deployed herein is not conducive to any conclusive statements on the issue of inequality regarding the difference in treatment between men and women. Gender issues are manifest in the practices traditionally associated with men and women. Although highly caricatured, two practices proved to be recurring sources of conflict and discreditation during consultations: first, driving in men and second, a concern and care for physical appearance in women.

Let us start with driving. Previously, geriatricians used to make their patient pass the "trail making test" in order to assess their ability to drive. Some of the patients fail, in which case it is "suggested" that they stop driving. Almost all of the men that I observed responded to such a suggestion either by promising to minimize the trips they made or by proclaiming and valuing their flawless behavior. For example, Mr. Duchesne exclaimed, "I put my blinker on every time! It's been forty years since I've been driving, and I'm putting my flashing on light every time. Forty years I've driven, and I've never forgotten to look in the rearview mirror. Uh, no . . . fifty years that I drive. Because I got my license at nineteen, you know." As we saw above, Mr. Dupond responded similarly.

The significance given to driving by men also appeared in my interview with Mr. Raulin, the former construction worker, and his wife. Mr. Raulin's wife constantly devalued him, repeating that he was "incapable," that he "doesn't know how to do anything," and so forth. Mr. Raulin, who seemed amorphous, almost never replied. Looking into the void, his head lowered and his jaw dangling, he muttered while his wife was talking. He probably abandoned the idea of being heard by anyone, except when I asked him why he never got his license. His wife answered on his behalf (as usual): "He is far too lazy. What'd you expect? He's bone idle!" Mr. Raulin suddenly raised his head and claimed with a surprisingly loud voice, "Hey! When I worked in construction, I was driving vehicles [he raises his arms], the wheels they were taller than me. So, d'you forget that? Well, then, bigger than me, the wheels! Well, then, the machines, they were twice the size of a car." Even those men who are most discredited do not abandon driving without resistance, or at the very least they cling to the memory of having previously maneuvered vehicles.

For elderly patients, driving is a condition of their material autonomy. Moreover, this form of material autonomy is closely related with driving's strong masculinist connotations. This symbolic association likely explains their reluctance to comply with the recommendations of the geriatricians in this respect, and yet, such reluctance to comply nevertheless entrenches their discreditation. Failing to comply with the geriatrician's "suggestion" means that they present as unreasonable people, affected by a disease that decreases the anticipation and perception of potential risks.

For women, refusals to appear stereotypically "elderly" and exhibit "old age" attributes, such as carrying a cane or wearing stockings, are considered inappropriate by doctors and relatives and therefore grounds for discreditation At the age of eighty-six, Mrs. Sauvignon, a former nursing aide, undertook this "caprice" with pride. In consultation, she exclaimed, "A cane? Never! It's for the little old ladies." After several falls, she would only compromise using a hiking stick found in her garage, which belonged to her nephew. The hiking stick resembled a walking stick but had a sharp metallic point at the tip. "With that, at least, I can defend myself!" she bragged when I visited her at her home. This compromise allowed her to justify the obedience to her doctors' and relatives' recommendations. However, it was not long until Mrs. Sauvignon's daughter replaced the metal peak (which slid on tiled surfaces) with a rubber tip and cut a part of the hiking stick to better fit Mrs. Sauvignon. The object no longer resembled anything even slightly threatening.

Ninety-two-year-old Mrs. Lopez also proclaimed her femininity by looking after her appearance. She came to consultations with conspicuous makeup, permanently curled hair dyed dark red, many jewels, chic clothes, a short skirt, and shoes with heels measuring about ten centimeters. Later her daughter informed us that she regularly fell at home because of the heels. This outfit discredited her right away and was the subject of regular conflicts in the family. The geriatrician suggested to Mrs. Lopez that her outfit and style were "no longer of [her] age." But, unsurprisingly, the patient did not respond to the incentives to stop wearing heels. The geriatrician also reprimanded her for her refusal to wear support stockings (compression stockings), attempting to procure an agreement by proposing in a playful voice, "You know, now there are stockings of all colors, and they are pretty." Mrs. Lopez responded with a pout of disgust. We also learned that Mrs. Lopez had undergone three cosmetic surgery operations. The geriatrician, in an obvious attempt to create complicity, commented in the same tone that one might use to conceal the blunder of a child, "That is our little secret!"

While female patients endeavor to maintain a "feminine" appearance, interpretations advanced in medical consultations do not consider this endeavor in such terms. The persistence of patients to maintain a "feminine" appearance produces a systematic discreditation. Like driving in men, the people around patients tend to interpret the behavior as the caprice of an old person affected by cognitive impairments.

Of Necessity and Spading: The Example of Mrs. Lefèvre

To go further in our exploration of discreditation, we must interrogate what these patterns of discreditation and their "latching effect" imply in the relation to others that discredited an individual's experience. My impression is that people suspected of or diagnosed with dementia tend to be continually in a position of justification because their situation is fundamentally devaluing for them.

This is how I interpret the tendency, among nursing home residents, to use the same techniques (recounting childhood memories, etc.) that I observed among the patients in memory consultations. Whoever their interlocutor is, they resort to these "lost talks." For example, Mrs. Jankevich, whom I met and interviewed in a French nursing home, tried to divert our conversation several times. When I questioned her about her daily life in the institution, she discussed her sense of being different—she was Jewish, and all the other residents were Catholics or atheists. She then took this topic as a way into a discussion about the history of her family, who were Polish immigrants deeply affected by the Second World War. She systematically reoriented the conversation toward the past. After one hour interviewing her about daily life in nursing home, I realized that I had learned nothing about the present.

Assuming that discredited people are constantly justifying themselves against their discreditation opens up certain avenues for interpreting their actions. The interview I conducted with Mrs. Lefèvre illustrates this particularly well. Mrs. Lefèvre is a seventy-eight-year-old former dental assistant who worked all her active life in Paris before settling in a house that she built with her siblings in the countryside, forty kilometers from the capital. She had two husbands; the last one was an accountant but died "some time ago." I met Mrs. Lefèvre through her case manager, a health professional called in event of an emergency to manage the domestic organization and caregiving network that surround complicated "cases." The village town hall called the case manager complaining of

Mrs. Lefèvre's "public drunkenness" and the ensuing "public disturbance." These difficulties necessitated the daily visit of a housekeeper. Moreover, Mrs. Lefèvre was no longer able to sustain independent living and would have to move to settle in her brother's house soon. Her daughter was present during the interview. She lived in New York but is temporarily back in France to rest after selling her business and is taking the opportunity to spend some time with her mother and take care of her.

We started the conversation in a very relaxed atmosphere. Leaning on a window while the patient and I sat around the living room table, Mrs. Lefèvre's daughter was able to indicate to me when she felt her mother was not telling the truth. She did this successfully without her mother noticing, sometimes with direct verbal disagreements. Mrs. Lefèvre exceled at reformulating situations to preserve the independence she claimed:

> *How did you meet Mrs. Meyer? [The case manager]*
> Mrs. L.: Oh, like that . . . maybe by chance! [Her daughter says no with her head, rolling her eyes] I cannot tell you exactly. It's been a while. I don't know anymore. Maybe at that time when we constructed the house, when there was the building permit to get, and she came by to see where the house will be. Or maybe when I had to launch the procedure for my retirement pension. Things like that. But when she's around, even if we have nothing to tell each other, she stops, she comes by the house. I sympathized with her, and she's pleasant.
> *So she comes by, time to time?*
> Mrs. L.: Yes, that's it. Her office is seven kilometers from here.
> *And are there any other professionals who come to see you, in addition to Mrs. Meyer?*
> Mrs. L.: Nobody else. I don't need anyone else. And even Mrs. Meyer, it's not a necessity, it's not an obligation, and she comes because we know each other.
> Daughter: There is also Cécile, who comes to help you.
> Mrs. L.: Yes, but Cécile is not the same. Cécile is my domestic help.
> D.: Yes, this is the question he's just asked you: is there someone who comes during the week to help you?
> Mrs. L.: Ah, okay, yeah, a little domestic help. She comes twice a week. Upon request, hey! If I ask her to come, she comes.
> *Does she come to do the housework or—*

Mrs. L.: Yes, or to do some grocery shopping, or, as I no longer drive and I don't want to spend money I don't have to buy another car, I take the opportunity to group all my activities and go in the car with her. I go with her.

You go . . . to do shopping with her?

Mrs. L.: Yeah. She's a very delightful woman.

It's that it's convenient—

Mrs. L.: But it's not indispensable!

[. . .]

And do you often see doctors?

Mrs. L.: Never! [Her daughter disagrees with a shake of her head] Except if, myself, I have to visit a doctor or somebody else . . . but by obligation, never.

D.: These days, you go there pretty often though, Mom.

Mrs. L.: Yes, but not by obligation.

D.: Well . . . yes, it's pretty much [obligatory].

Mrs. L.: We go there for X-rays or stuff like that, not obligatory things. . . . We do not go there because I don't eat or I don't sleep. . . . It's . . . it's mostly circulatory with me. I've always had blood issues.

D. [upset]: Mom, where were you yesterday?

Mrs. L.: Oh, you tire me! I don't know what we've done yesterday. I only know that the day has passed but . . . I don't know very well. . . . If I think of it, I could tell you. . . . Ah, doctors, fortunately, they exist. This is a fact. Because we . . .

Need them?

Mrs. L.: Yes, don't we? Don't we?

This excerpt shows how the patient uses rhetorical techniques in order to save face. When I questioned her about the professionals with whom she was in contact, she took me to be suggesting that they were "indispensable" or "compulsory." She implied that the help received was the secondary motivation of their visit. Above all, they would "occasionally" come by to "sympathize." It is difficult here to disentangle any cognitive disorders from the rest, which is to say that it is unclear when Mrs. Lefèvre forgot things and when she intentionally recalled only that which suited her.[14]

The conversation became quite tense when Mrs. Lefèvre explained that she would soon go to live with her brother and sell her house. In the first part of our interview, Mrs. Lefèvre praised the quality of her home and described how much she appreciated living in it. I initially regretted having asked her why she was going to move, fearing that she would feel trapped. However, my initial impression underestimated Mrs. Lefèvre's inexhaustible ability to redefine the situation:

> *Why are you going to leave? It's too complicated to stay here ... alone?*
> No, there is nothing complicated.
> *Okay ...*
> [Silence]
> I go to bed, I wake up. . . . There's no problem. I am a very orga-nized person who is not ... struggling. So ... my house is built, there is nothing to do there, I do not have to do new work. Me, I wake up ... it's a day like today, like it was yesterday. I am very organized, yes, I do not need anything, let's say ...
> Daughter: Mom ... [Intonation: be reasonable]
> Yes!
> [Silence]
> *And what are you going to do with this house?*
> Sell it. Yes, of course. With the money, I'll go ... hey, all my life I worked to earn money and to live with it, and then to make my life the best as I decided to, so now that I don't need anything anymore, I would like to discover what I could not know so far. [Silence. I feel that she and her daughter will argue if we continue]
> [...]
> *So there will be a little bit more people around you when you'll be there?*
> Oh yes! [Intonation expressing a carefree attitude] If I am around there, and if I go to the north of France where I have family too, I know that if I go in one place or another I would have a daily contact. . . . And as I have Magalie coming and having a car, friends coming and having a car ... my car, she no longer served me, and I was paying insurance for nothing. So I decided to dispose of it. But when I have to leave, when I'll go to my brother's, there I will buy a vehicle, there I will need one. [The daughter shakes her head, putting her hand on her head].

We can identify some of the techniques briefly mentioned above. For example, Mrs. Lefèvre insisted, again and again, that her house was well built. We can also note how she framed various daily situations so as to present herself as the decision-maker (especially concerning the sale of her car). And lastly, we can observe how she presented the move to her brother's house as a somewhat bohemian travel project that she devised after a hard life of sedentary work.

Because I conducted the interview as most sociologists do—nodding and encouraging the participant to keep talking—Mrs. Lefèvre's daughter seemed to worry, at a certain point, that I would believe her mother. At one point, she interrupted the conversation while Mrs. Lefèvre pretended to ignore this exchange. In such circumstances, I found myself caught in a discreditation configuration against my will. I was talking about Mrs. Lefèvre in front of her, all the while assuming that she did not understand everything that was said.

> D. (to me): Baptiste, what training did you do? Psychology?
> *No, I'm a sociologist.*
> D.: . . . Anyway, d'you have a sense of what's happening here?
> *Yeah, yeah.*
> D.: Ah, okay, good.

Paying attention to *social trajectories* may add further interpretive layers. During the interview, Mrs. Lefèvre put emphasis on her social belonging to the working class. Several times, she highlighted that she had worked all her life and that she had grown up in a workers' family. To indicate this affinity, she used the word *ouvrière* in a way that means "artisan," or at least "manual people": "We do a lot by ourselves." "I do everything by myself. I can tinker, get on the rooftops. I'm very manual. And that's why at the end of the day, when I could do reading, which is necessary for me, instead I go to bed right away." At the very least, Mrs. Lefèvre's voiced affinity with manual people offers a way to understand why she constantly extols the functional qualities of her house: "The house is small but very comfortable. Very well insulated. The walls are thick like that. We made it as a family, so it was made conscientiously, with appropriate materials. I do not use heating during the winter! I almost do not use heating. Yet I have heating everywhere. . . . It is small, it is not luxurious, but it is, say, functional."

In addition to the family building, Mrs. Lefèvre repeatedly associated herself with this "worker's" family tradition:

> *So, you read some newspapers too? [Looking at a newspaper laid on the table]*

Mrs. L.: Yes. Well, not systematically. It's not an obligation. When I don't know what to do I sit down and I read. . . . I'm not an intellectual, hey. I forgot to be one. I have what I need to live my life, because I worked, but apart from it . . . Not at all, I'm not an intellectual. I'm more the manual type. I spade, I sow seeds, I take care of the garden.
[Looking outside] You have some plants?
Mrs. L.: Well, there is some grass growing, and I don't have a lawnmower at the moment, it's broken. . . . My garden is my great neighbor. Oh, when I have my mower and my rake in my hands, nothing else matters to me.

Her daughter shook her head during this whole exchange. With a quick glance at the state of the garden, it was clear that Mrs. Lefèvre had not done gardening for some time. That said, Mrs. Lefèvre's subtle use of the present tense is notable. When she asserted, "I spade," she may have been referring to different uses of the term. It may have meant, variously, "I spade these days," "I spade in general" (not specifically yesterday or during the previous weeks), "I am more inclined to spade rather than read," or "I am the type of manual person who is more attached to her garden above all." Consequently, Mrs. Lefèvre's assertion can be understood as an attempt to provide a coherent picture of herself; or maybe she just thought that she had spaded recently.

Facing configurations of discreditation, sociologists must not strengthen the power relationship at work (by reinforcing the gestures, words, and practices of those who initiate the discreditation) nor uncritically give credence to discredited persons but open up possibilities for interpretation. We could take what Mrs. Lefèvre said as *symptoms*. In which case, she would be "in denial," not conscious that she receives professional help and that she regularly goes to the doctor, despite trying to "catch up" when her daughter reminded her of the "truth." However, such an interpretation would be hasty and judgmental, minimizing the value of her discourse and according all the credit to her case manager and her daughter. Alternatively, we could take what she said as *meanings*. According to this perspective, Mrs. Lefèvre would find herself in an intermediary situation where, while she received some caregiving, none of it would be strictly necessary. Yet such an interpretation is dismissive the views of her daughter and the case manager. It is also possible that Mrs. Lefèvre utilized various rhetorical techniques to save face, especially in front a stranger like me and in front of her daughter, who had the power to place her in a nursing home.

Another way to distance oneself from these questions of inter-pretation is to ask whether, in other situations, similar processes have been observed. During any research, the participants' percep-tion of their situation is expressed through "filters" pertaining to the particularities of the enunciation situation and their individual social trajectories. Participants try to answer questions in a way that does not jeopardize nor favor them. A good illustration can be found in the sociology of sexuality, where questionnaire sur-veys have long reported that women declare having had less sexual partners in their lifetimes than men. Facing the question "how many sexual partners have you had in your life?" researchers real-ized that men were inclined to count any sexual encounter while women selected only those sexual encounters with partners who were important to them; in other words, women who partook in questionnaires added a certain parameter to the question, namely the significance of the encounters.[15] Mrs. Lefèvre proceeded ac-cording to the same operation when she answered our questions by "filtering" them through her notion of necessity.

The Routinization of Discredit

As the previous interview illustrates, members of the family, at least those who are mobilized, concede a certain amount of credibility to their diagnosed relative, in the same way as doctors. However, they do so with different tools. Family members entertain a degree of credibility in order to establish which form of intervention is necessary, which would then enable the patient to live according to certain criteria. For example, when a person claims to be able to live alone or to be able to cook for himself or herself, the extent to which family members hear these claims *as credible* dramatically affects the different support devices that might be established. As is the case in consultations, the discovery of any discrepancy between words and actions (between saying one thing, such as "I cook for myself," and appearing emaciated) increases the likelihood of being discredited. In the attempt to anticipate domestic and health risks, people are discredited.

Family members sometimes disagree on the amount of credibility to be accorded to the patient. In this regard, placement in a nursing home is a time of increased tension because, in many cases, family members decide on placement against the will of the placed person. The family's reasoning is typically as follows: if an individual speaks of a "will" to stay at home, for instance, and if their words are not considered sufficiently credible, then these words cannot be justifiably considered a manifestation of the "will." Mr. Lautrec found himself in this situation and testified in his diary:

> June 14th, 9pm. Fell over in my room with Grandma [his wife]
>
> 11PM Emergency services called. They finally come. Put Grandma back to bed and keep me. At 0:30 am, dropped at emergency clinic
>
> I will never go back to my home where I lived for 36 years
>
> June 17th, shoulder brooch.
>
> June 18th. Josianne [his daughter] comes from Rennes, takes care of everything. In a state of physical and moral incapacity, I have been abused. For a long time, they wanted me to look as an Alzheimer, to decide for me.

The reasons that lead individuals to give credit to the patients or, on the contrary, to evaluate the risks of believing them are multiple and particularly acute in times of crisis. These reasons largely involve the availability and endurance of family caregivers. If all family caregivers say, at the beginning of the illness trajectory, that it is out of the question to place their relative in a nursing home, few actually succeed in doing so when managing the troubles requires an investment in terms of time, money, and "energy" that they can no longer provide.

The intervention of professionals (which is linked to the family's estimation of the patient's situation and the various management options) can then change the game. When Mrs. Lavoie was hospitalized after a fall, she and her husband, both diagnosed with early stage dementia, considered themselves capable of staying at home. Worried, the couple's children intervened and initiated a procedure to place them in a nursing home. The children no longer believed what their parents said, or at least considered that believing them would be too dangerous. A social worker then acted in support of Mr. and Mrs. Lavoie staying home. They discussed this episode during our interview:

SOCIAL WORKER: [To Mrs. Lavoie] Do you remember when we first met at the hospital? There was a fall . . . then they [children] said you had memory problems, then you had to give up your driver's license, and then . . . I noticed that your children often told you what to do. Then you got very angry—

MR. LAVOIE: Very angry, yeah.

MRS. LAVOIE: It still upsets me. . . .

SW: But you still have help every morning to take your drugs . . .

MRS. LAVOIE: Yeah, but I can't wait to finish because I'm sick of taking them!

SW: But here you are autonomous. Apart from that, you are autonomous. But do your children tell you what to do?

MR. LAVOIE: No, no. Well, from time to time they will suggest—

MRS. LAVOIE: They will suggest—

MR. LAVOIE: They will suggest this or that thing . . . [. . .]

SW: Then you, how do you react to that?

MR. LAVOIE: Oh, it doesn't bother us, but we tell them . . . "Go work instead!" [. . .] There is no one who'll lead us. No one.

[Mr. Lavoie speaks of his youth, when his parents "already" had difficulties telling him what to do]

Some devices formalize discredit, including guardianship. The person under guardianship is formally deprived of the right to make decisions regarding the management of their bank accounts, the care they receive, and possibly their institutionalization. Beyond practical issues, having to ask someone else to make even the smallest purchase, to make the slightest decision, is experienced as a humiliating situation. Mrs. Vanin said that as a former worker, living under guardianship was an offense to her trajectory. She felt this offense particularly acutely because she received money as if she needed financial assistance. Mrs. Vanin felt as if she had not earned this money by herself: "I always have a little bit of money because when he [her nephew/guardian] comes, he brings me some. But I don't know, that's a set of things. I don't feel alive. Actually, it's difficult to explain, but I've always worked a lot, a lot.

For the members of the family or, if there is no family, for the professionals who decide to put patients under guardianship, the issue is above all a matter of "protection." Indeed, the people I met under guardianship occasionally faced accusations of unreasonable spending. Patients faced accusations of "inordinate" tips or purchases of "unnecessary" items. On the matter of alleged financial "mismanagement," it must be said that there is a flourishing business of swindling the elderly. From workers who illegally offer overpriced services to commercially lawful companies who take advantage of elderly customers by selling them everything they can, aged persons face many threats from supposedly legitimate goods and service providers. People living under guardianship experience this situation as a questioning of their whole trajectory, as a negation of their efforts to provide for themselves during their entire life.

In the media and in public policies, tensions associated with the discredit process are publicized, principally, as a moral attitude—that is, as an ethical behavior toward illness and the elderly. As far as possible, the opinions of those affected individuals should be taken into consideration, in respect of their autonomy as individuals. In practice, though, it is mainly a matter of conflicting estimations regarding the risks associated with the diagnosed person. The result is a dissatisfaction that is difficult to circumvent. Patients often complain that they have been deprived of their rights, and family members often regret that they were not able to provide the necessary care for their loved one in a more consensual way. In the case of professionals involved in the discreditation process, they are often aware that they propose the "least bad" solution. Most of the actors involved in the process consider their actions a necessary evil. The widely consulted recommendations available online for families and professionals do not change anything. They highlight the necessity of gauging the "level of aptitude" of the diagnosed persons in order to best accommodate them in the decision-making processes.

Finally, when discreditation is total or almost total, interlocutors consider that patients are no longer aware of the interactions they experience or that such awareness is minimal. Therefore, interlocutors regard it as futile to envisage the development of a relationship with the patient according to all the usual social codes. Discreditation is routinized.

Most interlocutors thus consider it preferable to refrain from communicating information to the discredited persons regarding the state of their health or the situation in which they find themselves. It is better, one supposes, to spend quality time with the patient and not to worry about such matters.

MRS. LOPEZ (SERIOUS): I have a question.

DOCTOR: Yes, Mrs. Lopez.

MRS. L.: Am I already crazy?

D. (LAUGHING): Don't worry, you're not crazy. At ninety-two, we can't be crazy at this age!

Discredited persons are then included in the exchanges, but in a peripheral manner, in much the same fashion that children are peripherally included in "adult" discussions. That is to say, they make comments that are heard without being integrated into the fabric of the conversation. This sort of peripheral inclusion occurred when I conducted an interview with Mr. Raulin and his wife. It is a tendency I failed to reverse during the course of our exchange:

> *So you got married a long time ago?*
> Mr. Raulin (very low, quietly): It was, it was a few years ago now. . . .
> Mrs. Raulin (at the same time, louder): It was in 1994.
> *Ah, yes, twenty years! What's the wedding anniversary for this?*
> Mr. R. (very low): I think it's—

Mrs. R. (at the same time, louder): Yes, twenty years. We will soon celebrate the porcelain wedding!

Mr. R. (laughing, very low): Hahah, yes, porcelain, porcelain.

And you have children?

Mr. R. (very low): Not with . . .

Mrs. R. (at the same time, louder): No, well, yes, but from another marriage.

The interactions increasingly resemble a game, with the aim of only "passing the time," to entertain, and not to exchange information, opinions, or news. What is said and expressed is intended only to manage the present moment.

Conclusion

The social experience of dementia is a progressive experience of discreditation. In order to understand how this characteristic relates to a certain social context in more detail, let us pose, speculatively, the following question: what social conditions would be necessary in order that the words and behaviors of the diagnosed persons are not solely interpreted through the prism of their cognitive disorders? *What would it take* for other interpretations to exist? I offer four hypotheses in response to this question.

The first hypothesis is that, in our societies, the only interpretative prism regarding patients' discourse is medical theory, according to which neurological and bodily disorders lead people to experience a distorted perception of reality. Not only is this framework dominant, because doctors have a determining institutional and cultural power, but it is increasingly the only one available.[16] The extent of this monopolization with respect to interpretive frameworks explains the difficulties often encountered when one tries to give the words of the diagnosed persons a meaning other than "symptomatic." These attempts are often heard as radical, unfounded, and far-fetched.

The second hypothesis is a corollary of the first. If the only interpretation framework available is medical, it is because there are no social actors or organizations sufficiently influential to disseminate others. Let us take the world of work as an example. There, many "ambiguous" behaviors are observable. Workers sometimes perform non-work-related activities in their workplaces, deliberately slow down the pace of production, or declare themselves sick to avoid coming to the office when they have no signs of physical illness.[17] From these behaviors, several interpretations are possible. Often, the people in charge of the companies consider the behaviors to be the result of laziness or individual irresponsibility. However, most trade unions see such behaviors as signs of resistance to unacceptable working conditions. Discussions of suicide in the workplace highlight these divergences. Some believe that workers commit suicide in their workplaces because they suffer from individual vulnerability. For others, it would be the consequence of the misdeeds of the organization itself. If there are several interpretations, it is because a long history of theoretical frameworks (managerial theories, Marxist criticisms of labor, etc.) carried by conflicting organizations has rendered such interpretations possible.[18] These interpretive frameworks vary according to place and culture. It is well known, for example, that in France the trade union interpretation is more widely diffused than elsewhere. While comparison between interpretations of cognitive disorder and labor has its limits, it nevertheless allows us to note that in the field of aging and dementia, there is no such history. There have been no social movements strong enough to produce alternative interpretations of the patients' behavior.

The third hypothesis is a further corollary. The medical model places elderly patients in a structurally unfavorable situation because of the values contained with the model. As we have seen, a patient is judged by professionals and members of the family in accordance with the patient's cognitive performance. It is an expectation that patients will remember the things they have just done, that they ensure that their words are consistent with their practices, and so on. However, as people age, cognitive performance diminishes, and, facing the threat of being placed in nursing homes (or any other form of dispossession of their daily lives), older people tend to exaggerate their capacity to live at home without help. In

sum, older people are *structurally disadvantaged by the social criteria used for assessing them.*

As always, we study other cultures to think ours is useful. In
a Native American community in Oklahoma,[19] anthropologists
observed that certain symptoms suggestive of an advanced stage
of dementia, such as "delusions," acquire a mystical interpretation.
In these cases, approaching death means being able to see what is
"on the other side." Harriet G. Rosenberg observed that among the
Ju/'hoansi in Botswana,[20] the help provided to the elderly is valued
to such an extent that it is not perceived as a favor but as a duty
for which no gratitude has to be expressed. Even when they live
in good conditions, elders constantly complain to maintain pressure on their family and a position of power in the community.
By complaining, pressure is applied in order to remind others in
the group that it is the right of the elder to demand the best care
possible. These examples show that cognitive performance is not
a "natural" or "obvious" criterion for assessing the credibility of
older people but that our medicalized conception of aging tends to
establish these cultural criteria, specific to our society and our history, as the only possible ones.

The fourth hypothesis is, again, a further corollary. There is
no ritual allowing diagnosed persons to express their opinions in a
legitimate way. Consider the following example: When the citizens
of a country vote, regardless of their political positions, from the
moment they go to the polling stations show their voters' cards,
enter the polling booths, and perform all the ritual steps of vot-
ing, their votes will be counted. Put differently, the content of a
voter's opinion does not determine its consideration; rather, it is
respect of the ritual that governs its expression. We cannot imagine
a polling station where only votes that express a supposedly "reasonable" opinion, according to those responsible for organizing the
vote, would be admissible. Yet, in a way, this is precisely what happens with discredited individuals: their interlocutors consider their
opinions on a case-by-case basis, according to what they deem
reasonable and plausible. There is no ritual framework enabling

patients to express their opinions, which would enable them to be taken seriously.

In other words, thus far I have attempted to demonstrate the way in which the experience of dementia is an experience of discredit; I herein suggest that this type of interaction pattern is made possible, structurally, by the absence of theories, actors, movements, institutions, and rituals capable of producing other possibilities and alternative interpretations.

3

THE DEFERENCE INDUSTRY

SINCE THE MIDTWENTIETH CENTURY, THERE HAS BEEN A sharp increase in services aimed at caring for the elderly, and this process has been accompanied by the intensified production of moral discourses seeking to define the ideal modes of behavior to be used in relation to these persons. A whole arsenal of expressions, words, and images draw a line between good and evil, between what should be done and not done.

This *moralization of care* has emerged in response to the previously substandard hospitals where psychiatric patients, elderly persons, and other destitute or marginalized populations were confined. The idea was to replace asylums with welcoming, specialized, warm institutions where the patients receive "humane" treatment. As an increasing public health priority in most Western countries, Alzheimer's disease and related dementias were the subject of large awareness campaigns, spearheaded by public authorities and the media. Subsequently, the dissemination of public health campaigns contributed to the growth of these moral discourses in all types of service.

As one moves through the health-care world, this "humanization movement" appears omnipresent, like a benevolent force behind the radiant faces, sparkling smiles, grateful glances, and intertwined hands that populate the promotional brochures of home assistance services and residences for seniors. This imagery provides professionals with an ideal representation of what they can do "well" despite their often difficult working conditions. In one of the institutions I observed, colleagues and managers described an extremely involved nursing aide's behavior as an "example to follow":

> "Mr. Roger, are you okay?" The staff member wears a big smile, tilting her head slightly, and places her hand on the resident's arm. The resident mumbles something. The caregiver gives me a look of complicity and then tilts more so that her gaze is at the same level as the patient's—a frequent recommendation in good behavior guides with patients suffering from dementia. She smiles even more, eyes wide open, expressing attention, compassion. "You look good today." Her words are clearly articulated, and her voice is clear, soft, and slightly sharper in pitch than the one she uses with her colleagues. She strokes the arm of patient, who stares at the floor. "Well, I'm leaving you."

The humanist discourses avowed by many professionals—"I like to work with people," "this job is like a gift," and so on—resonate with the official discourse of health systems, which is illustrated well by the code of ethics displayed on the walls of a Montreal institution: "We believe that human beings are constantly evolving and that they do so, until the end of their life, no matter their condition. For us, each person is unique. We believe in the potential, the strengths, and the capacity of each individual to support themselves, alone or with the support of their relatives."

The humanization movement gives rise to a polarization of values and images. A set of words embodies the positive pole: ill people remain "human beings," "persons" having the "right" to be treated "decently," with "respect," "benevolence," "dignity," and "good treatment."[1] The other side of the discourse takes the form of global condemnation of abuse against the elderly, carried out at the international level by the United Nations and the World Health Organization.

Thus, the moment someone appears to suffer from a form of dementia, the interlocutors with whom she or he is led to interact entertain this particular humanist ideal, or at least they are "exposed" to this polarization of conduct between good and evil, between human and inhuman, between good treatment and abuse. In this chapter, I will analyze this dimension of the social experience of dementia but in terms of *deference*.

Critique of the Uses of Humanity as a Value

My choice to use the concept of deference primarily stems from a critique of humanistic discourses in dementia care. Humanistic discourses explain that it is by virtue of their "humanity" or "humanness," because they are "persons," that diagnosed patients are to be treated "humanely." Humanistic discourses appeal to a common humanity, blind to racial, gender, and class determinations. By virtue of this common humanity, patients are entitled to benefit from a certain type of behavior (namely, that employees greet them, are polite, etc.) and a certain type of material framework (namely, sleeping in a clean place, eating appropriately, etc.).

From a public policy point of view, a certain amount of money will be spent and a set of measures taken to promote this "human" treatment of "human" users in health-related services, such as home care companies and nursing homes. With this in mind, health facilities in the Quebec sector must comply with a number of formalized standards, mostly decreed by Accreditation Canada (an independent agency) and the minister of Health and Social Services. These standards aim to express the values mentioned above: [Extract from a minister's working document] "Indeed, respect for the dignity and rights of the resident is to be reflected in courteous and amiable interventions. . . . A relational approach, gentle, warm, and benevolent ensures a quality of the presence during the exchanges between the employees, the resident, and their caregiver. Respect for privacy in commonplaces, as well as written and verbal confidentiality about the resident, are also necessary to ensure respect for the dignity and rights of the resident."

For its part, management of the institutions seek to define objectives in line with these values and to redefine them as assessable indicators.

> [Working document of a facility observed in Quebec]
> Relationship with the client: this indicator concerns the relationship between the staff and the users. This relationship is humanistic and based on respect for the person and his / her rights. . . .
> Respect: consideration that a person deserves because of the human value that we recognize in them and which leads us to behave towards them with reserve and restraint. Respect involves discreet

behavior in an environment careful of the user's privacy. Respect also underpins the acceptance of difference.

Professionals working at different levels within the institution translate these values into the terms that reflect their reality. Thus, this manager insists on the "satisfaction" of the residents, regularly measured by surveys conducted among residents and then interpreted as an indicator of the quality of the services provided by the facility: "The relational aspect is the most important thing. In order for a resident to be satisfied with our services, to be happy in his or her environment, what influences his or her satisfaction the most is the quality of the relationship that the staff members will have with him or her. How residents will feel respected, recognized as human beings."

Let us take a step back. What is meant by "humanity" in these humanistic discourses? We can shed light on this question by comparing how states deal with different publics. An array of people of different social status are being treated in an array of different ways, with humanity given a multivalent set of connotations. Senior officials do not receive the same level of care as homeless people, and different rules of decorum apply to nursing home residents, prisoners of war, and foreign diplomats. Yet all are human, and in many cases their humanity is taken as a core value by the host organizations. Thus, article 13 of the Geneva Convention stipulates "prisoners of war must be treated at all times with humanity." In September 2012, the European Court of Justice defined "religious persecution" as meaning an actual risk of "being prosecuted or subjected to inhuman or degrading treatment or punishment"; the victims of these practices can be welcomed in Europe with refugee status. Even seals are concerned: the European Parliament, when it decided to set up an embargo on products derived from seal hunts, argued that this hunt is "inhuman."

What is defined as human in each case does not imply the same standards or the same cost. The relevant matter, then, is not whether people *are* humans but how, under cover of a generalized notion of "humanity," some enjoy a certain *social status* befitting the allocation of certain material means and the receipt of certain behaviors while others do not.[2] What is at issue here, in particular, is the receipt of *deference*.

Erving Goffman draws attention to the notion of deference, which, on his account, lays the very foundation for social interactions. As a key feature of the ground for social interaction, deference denotes that through which individuals perform and realize social stratification on a daily basis. Goffman speaks of deference as "that component of activity which functions as a symbolic means by which appreciation is regularly conveyed to a recipient of this recipient, or of something of which this recipient is taken as a symbol, extension, or agent."[3] Put simply, when you interact with someone, part of your behavior visibly expresses recognition of the other's social status. When you call your doctor "Doctor," for example, or when you tuck your children in bed and kiss them before they sleep, greet your boss with some respect, or even give cute nicknames to your spouse, you show them that they receive this attention because they hold a specific status. They are your doctor, your children, your boss, or your spouse. Take all of these behaviors, and you grasp what Goffman calls deference.

Importantly, Goffman's notion of deference allows us to study how differences between social groups manifest in ordinary interactions. Beyond this, the notion of deference assists us in questioning the political and social issues involved in these interactions. It is not insignificant, for example, that the title "miss" (*mademoiselle*) is now officially removed from the French language and that officials in communist countries referred to each other as "comrade." Governing formal appellations that express social statuses supposedly fosters egalitarianism between genders and social classes, respectively. Unsurprisingly, whom the recipient of deference is, how deference is claimed, and through which symbolism are political matters.

An equally significant dimension of deference is expressed in a more discreet and unconscious manner through everyday life attitudes, intonations, and gestures. This raises equally political questions, as Alexis de Tocqueville already noted during his visit to the United States at the beginning of the nineteenth century:

> In aristocratic communities where a small number of persons manage everything, the outward intercourse of men is subject to settled conventional rules. Everyone then thinks he knows exactly what marks of respect or of condescension he ought to display, and none are presumed to be ignorant of the science of etiquette. . . .
>
> But as the distinctions of rank are obliterated, as men differing in education and in birth meet and mingle in the same places of resort, it is almost impossible to agree upon the rules of good breeding. . . . There are many little attentions which an American does not care about; he thinks they are not due to him, or he presumes that they are not known to be due: he therefore either does not perceive a rudeness or he forgives it; his manners become less courteous, and his character more plain and masculine.[4]

Tocqueville explains that in societies where a democratic and/ or egalitarian political system is in place, where "ranks fade" (in appearance at least), it becomes impossible to regulate interactions with the same precision as within an aristocratic social order. Hence the impression that courtesy disappears and manners are deregulated, since all citizens would be statutorily equal. But Tocqueville, like some present-day observers, yields too quickly to his first impressions. In our societies, behind the apparent informality of relations, and behind the egalitarianism displayed, status-related norms persist and orientate social relations. The difference is that they are less planned, less codified, rapidly evolving, and less obvious to understand. This relative contradiction between equality (showing that we are equal) and distinction (showing, even if we do not intend to, that we belong to unequal groups) creates a crucial tension in contemporary social life.

In this fashion, the "humanist" discourse insists on the egalitarian dimension of the deference produced toward the elderly. Everyone is human, it says, and as humans, patients are entitled to care. However, in practice, it is not their biological "humanity" that entitles them to such deference; it is rather on account of their particular status that they receive these marks of "humanity." This is because, among other things, elderly people diagnosed with dementia constitute a social group considered vulnerable. They are labeled with a diagnosis that is constitutive of a public health priority, and this disease does not involve any socially prejudicial behavior. We did not observe the same hastiness to label as "humans" the first people diagnosed with HIV.

The humanization movement toward the elderly living with dementia can be considered a set of initiatives aiming to change the standards of deference toward them by offering them a treatment perceived as more "appropriate" with respect to their social status. In view of the human and financial resources involved in these initiatives, and their embeddedness into a globalized sector of activity, it is no exaggeration to speak of dementia care as a veritable *industry of deference.*[5]

The Spontaneist Conception of Deference

In nursing homes, medical-related practices such as distributing medicines, hospitality practices such as serving meals, and all apparently "peripheral" contact such as corridor discussions realize this perceived right of the residents to receive a certain attention— *deference*. In this context, staff members carry out—and are expected to operate—a permanent staging of their benevolence. This staging occurs through words, intonations, gestures, facial expressions (for example, not having a "closed face"), and a disposition to "convert" moments of physical presence into conversations, even physical contact or visual exchanges.

Interactions between professionals and residents can occur at the time of prescribed tasks:

> A staff member distributes juices at snack time. She asks residents if they prefer apple, orange, or pineapple juice. She starts talking with one of them. "Mr. Rambeau, how are you? Did you watch your TV show today?" She puts a glass close to him. "No, I was chatting in the hall! Guess what, I found some companionship!" She goes to see another resident.
>
> When an employee comes to pick up a resident in her room to take her to an activity, the employee finds the resident reading the newspaper. "Is the news good, Mrs. Letang?" The resident laughs, "Oh! They bore me with their stories!"

Alternatively, interactions between professionals and residents can emerge from unplanned interactions, especially when employees have nothing specific to do, except to ensure the safety of the residents.

> A nursing assistant approaches a resident. She gently sits next to her, smiling, and addresses her while touching her arm. "So, Ms. Bobillard, are you okay?" The resident moans. She apparently agrees. The nursing assistant smiles more insistently. "Your vest is beautiful! Did your daughter give it to you?" "No, I . . . kni . . . kni . . . " "Did you knit it?" The resident nods. "Well done!" the nursing assistant exclaims before leaving.
>
> A nursing assistant is looking for a board game in the hall. Incidentally, she touches the shoulder of a resident with her hand and redirects the chair of another one who was watching television askew.

In the army, some codes explicitly govern the treatment a person is entitled to receive given their status.[6] Generals do not receive the same attention as sergeants, and the forms of attention received is prescribed by military rules. There is a protocol, no matter to what extent soldiers wish to follow it. The contrary takes place in nursing homes. Rather than observing explicit rules, the spontaneity of the produced attentions is most valued. Not only do the employees have to respect the existing codes (politeness and benevolence staging, for example), but in addition they must demonstrate sincerity in their interactions with patients. Indeed, to appear mechanical in one's staging of deference would be problematic. This *spontaneist conception of deference* strongly permeates the discourse of all nursing home actors, from managers and employees to residents themselves.

According to the residents, what makes a good employee is not only professionalism but also the way employees behave with them. That is to say, attributes displaying such congenial behavior include how employees chat with residents, serve meals, and greet them and the extent to which the employees are able to create pleasant conversations perceived as informal. Mrs. Corbin, an eighty-nine-year-old former shopkeeper who resides in a French nursing home, spoke of a trainee who had just come by her room: "You see, her,

Evelyne, that's her name, she was knitting with me just over here [in her room]. It's probably her time off." This was not Evelyne's time off but rather work time when she did not have any pressing task to accomplish. Employees are encouraged to socialize with residents during these times. For residents, receiving such visits or having conversations on these occasions is perceived as a rewarding form of attention, precisely because employees seem to choose to come and see them, as if spontaneously.

Staff members also value their work by placing emphasis on its human dimension. Most staff members recount that they like "relational" work, and those staff members occupying a professional tier (nursing assistants especially) consider that this relational aspect gives meaning to their routine. Regardless of whether their work is physically and mentally difficult, as well as poorly paid, staff members say that this work enriches them on a human level. A nurse explained, "When I go home and think . . . that maybe I have done something to improve, a little, that I gave a smile, gave a little happiness to an elderly person . . . [smile] well . . . I made my day." This satisfaction is often associated with a personality trait, something that has been there for a long time, as a nursing assistant commented: "I've always loved to take care of people. . . . I'm like that, so I'm here!"

While staff members have a set of relatively technical tasks to accomplish, such as giving food to residents or waking them up in the morning, they conceive of what is "noble" in their work in terms of what they do *in addition to* the basic prescribed tasks.[7] The exemplary nursing assistant mentioned above embodies this form of commitment: such an assistant is effective in doing the necessary tasks and is particularly active during and between each of these tasks, taking the opportunity to converse with the residents, not hesitating to hold and embrace them (unlike more distant colleagues), and organizing activities beyond the demands of their prescribed tasks. This "personal," "spontaneous," and even physical involvement ultimately constitutes a source of valorization.

For the executives of these institutions, the spontaneist conception of deference necessitates a certain type of personnel management. This is what emerges from my conversations with the director of the facility studied in France. On several occasions, he shared with me his concern to hire employees who have, in addition to technical skills, "the desire to work with humans." If all nurses have hospital training and therefore know how to provide the necessary physical care, these skills do not suffice. According to him, it is necessary to have a "common sense" inclination, among other things, to contribute to the life of the institution during idle times. He told me that he had difficulty finding enough employees who meet this criterion. He also explains the subtlety demanded in the management of such a facility. For example, "over-controlling" the employees, obliging them to behave in a certain way with the residents, is counterproductive. Such control threatens to undermine the atmosphere of the institution, precisely because the benevolence (deference) produced can no longer emerge "spontaneously." This mode of management can be described, to borrow Lopez's formula, as "organized emotional care."[8]

The Backstage of Deference

The deference produced "spontaneously" is in fact subject to control. We have seen that beyond the observed institutions, many political, health, local, national, and international actors are involved in the production of deference standards toward the elderly—a mobilization that many other social groups are not subject to. From local health centers to the United Nations, an incalculable set of actors seeks to define what constitutes appropriate behavior in this area. Moreover, within nursing homes, evaluation of the deference produced determines the very existence of a facility and of the work collective. Indeed, if a staff member is considered insufficiently pleasant with the residents, their managers might blame them or even fire them. If evaluations suggest that a facility is failing to treat its residents with all the "necessary" consideration, its director may be fired, the facility may be closed, or it may be placed under guardianship.

One characteristic of this control is its highly *external* character. Not all industries are subject to external control or intervention regarding deference production. Consider banks and nightclubs, for instance: no external institution seeks to regulate the politeness of the bankers or nightclub barmen except in some legal cases, for example, of discrimination. On the contrary, the nursing home sector is characterized by strong external control, since many actors *outside* these institutions attempt to influence the way in which the interactions occur *inside* them. The accreditations required for a facility to be authorized to operate require "evidence" that the residents benefit from a "quality" relational environment. Some public debates relayed by the media and certain political actors focus on this environment and its standards. Families and residents' committees also tend to give their opinions. It is therefore not surprising that this control of the deference produced emerges through a moral perspective. This is likely because these external actors must show that they operate on the basis of "higher imperatives" to justify their intervention.

Various forms of *internal* control follow. First, employees are often observed by their colleagues, managers, and residents or their families, since most of their tasks take place in the presence of others. This is not a control device as such. However, when a problem is reported (for example, a resident's relative complains about some treatment, an executive reports the inappropriate behavior of a nurse, etc.), each can testify to what they saw and what they consider appropriate. When new employees arrive in an institution, the executives usually ask older staff members what they think of their character. The rest of the time, executives assess the satisfaction of relatives and residents, either by formal surveys or by more informal means, such as discussions during their regular visits in the residents' rooms.

Interactions between staff members and residents partly build the "ambiance" of a facility, an atmosphere to which most residents and their families are sensitive and that plays a crucial role in their appreciation of the quality of the services. This atmosphere therefore becomes an *object of management*.

In some facilities, managers ask their employees to take their downtime (periods of relative inactivity) as opportunities to organize activities with residents and to set up these activities in common rooms, leaving the doors open. In this way, not only do residents feel that the professionals spontaneously offer activities to them, since they are unplanned activities, but the result is quickly visible. Three employees playing board games with a few residents in a public place conveys a very lively image to families who visit their relatives. In one of the institutions observed, music was also broadcast in the lobby, where several residents gathered. When I realized that very few people heard the music because of their hearing problems, a manager explained to me that this sound environment was intended mainly for families. With this device, they were more likely to have a positive feeling about the institution right from the entrance. In fact, the recipient of deference is not always the person who receives it. In other words, deference can be expressed toward someone (a resident) such that another person (a family member) notices it.

This whole setup also constitutes a form of control. Not only does the family's satisfaction contribute to the success of a facility (even if they generally do not have much choice due to the market situation), but mandatory industry evaluations also determine a facility's reputation. In Quebec, the evaluations of the Ministry of Health and Social Services and Accreditation Canada combine over two thousand standards. These standards concern safety, medication, material framework, care, behavior, and professionals' knowledge. These agencies visit each facility, rate it, and provide recommendations for improvement. The received score becomes part of the facility's reputation. To address these recommendations, executives then compose working groups with various professionals. These working groups must put in place measures to convince the evaluators that the problem identified has been resolved. Of course, this is until the next evaluation, where new weaknesses will be observed.

Assessments therefore generate practical changes within institutions. A few years before my research, gaps in the meal service had been identified in one of the observed facilities:

> [A manager] Several aspects were pointed out: equipment, having benches at the right height, having height-adjustable tables also, which would enable the resident to be well positioned, also regarding

the relational approach, naming what the resident will eat, saying the menu, serving dish after dish, respecting the residents' rhythm. So, first we made a video that was shown to all employees, to show the right technique. Then we developed a tool to list what the employee should do, and then, afterwards, the managers of each unit observe their employees and offer feedback. It is a process of continuous improvement.

And that was in response to ministerial visits?

Yes, yes, it was also to know what to tell them when they'd ask us, "What did you do to improve it?"

Note that the video in question was titled "The Privilege of Laying the Table." The expression is eloquent. It illustrates perfectly the relationship between the humanization of services and the social status of residents, which is thus "enhanced," at least symbolically, by a "noble" vocabulary. The video would certainly have seemed less distinguished if it had been named "The Joy of Setting the Table" or "The Pleasure of Serving a Meal."

Each actor converts the abstract values of humanization into technical or behavioral norms. Here are some excerpts from a working document redacted by a working committee set up after a ministerial visit:

- The menu is displayed daily
- The menu is explained verbally to the resident at meal times
- An alternative to the menu and choices are offered to the resident if the need arises
- The resident's food requirements and particularities are recorded in the work plan
- The entire team is present at meal times
- The delivery time of the food trolley conforms to the time determined by the food service
- Staff are waiting to be ready to feed the resident before placing the tray in front of him/her
- The temperature of the dishes is adequate and verified
- The presentation of the meal is attractive
- Staff provide adequate vigilance and assistance in all places where residents eat
- Benches or chairs at the correct height are available and used by staff

- Recreation staff consult the residents' life histories to personalize activities
- Staff explain their interventions beforehand to the residents
- Staff knock on the door before entering a residents' room, after waiting for a response
- Staff announce their name and present themselves when they enter a resident's room
- Staff exchange with resident during care
- Staff do not socialize with each other during the care given to the resident.

This list provides a series of regulations for employees and also serves as a rubric for executives circulating in the facility, in order to observe and evaluate employees' work practices. "You forgot to announce the menu there. Will you try to do it next time?" "You were not really at the same height as the patient. You have to be at the same level." Such individual evaluations proceed on a regular basis. Executives observe interactions in order to gauge whether the employee performs each of the listed gestures. For managers, the acquisition of new standards is established on the basis of norms that must be said and repeated. "[Interview with an executive] As a priority here, we decide to meet on day, evening, and night shifts to always talk to them [the employees] about the importance of being in touch with the resident. So we try to create, I will tell you by repeating, repeating, repeating to the employees, 'Do not forget to be in touch with the resident!' And also I've always thought if the employees are happy, the residents will be. So I try to also work to tell the employees when they are doing the right things."

In addition to evaluations, some executives try to initiate team-by-team change processes. A Quebec manager recounted how she asked each team to take on a challenge. Giving oneself a challenge, rather having a challenge imposed by another, helps to cultivate the "spontaneity" necessary to the deference produced.

> For one team the task was to improve the atmosphere during the snack time. So instead of going into each room to give the yogurts or anything, making sure to create an atmosphere at that time. For the

other team, it was teamwork, not keeping information but sharing, especially life stories, say for example, "You know with Mrs. so-and-so, don't do this with her. You're gonna make her aggressive for the rest of the day. Do it like this instead." There was this unit that had chosen to make sure that all the celebrations were highlighted by decoration. So they crafted themes to make the environment pleasant, and then they involved the residents. It may be trivial, but it changes everything. In each team there is a board with the challenges marked. It is not me or the manager of the unit that chooses.

All these processes give rise to labor-intensive writing and archiving. I have never been able to count the number of binders containing the employees' activity reports. Every day I discovered a new binder, not to mention the digitized records kept on the associated online platforms. Everything is noted, printed, and classified, and most improvement initiatives give rise to new sheets to fill out. For assessment agencies, no written record is beyond the scope of evaluation. As a result, the time professionals spend on administrative tasks increases. In Quebec, nurses have reclaimed responsibility for many of these tasks and, in recent years, have acquired an increasingly administrative role while disengaging themselves from clinical tasks. They have delegated these clinical tasks to nursing assistants while delegating hygiene-related tasks to nursing aides. In this organization, nurses have also had to assume roles as team manager. Because of this changing division of labor, paralleled with workforce reductions, nursing aides have seen the scale of their work increase dramatically.

Despite being aware of these expanding workplace responsibilities and the accompanying acceleration of work rhythms, managers emphasize a positive aspect. According to them, the rise of service improvement programs and "tools" set up to implement these programs (formalizing them in written form) improved the overall quality of the services provided. The "relational quality" of care is now more *uniform* because it is formalized by written protocols that can circulate between units and more *controllable* because evaluable.

As we have now seen, the deference production in nursing homes is characterized simultaneously by its spontaneist conception, its strong external control, and its increasing bureaucratization.

Relational Techniques in Deference Production

However, the standards structuring deference in nursing homes obviously do not encapsulate the issues raised by deferential activities throughout interactions. During my fieldwork, I found it very difficult to adopt a posture that seemed "satisfactory" toward the residents. Here, *satisfactory* refers to the subjective adequacy between a form of deference produced and the social status of its recipient. How should one take into consideration the difficulties faced by each resident? How should one react in unforeseen situations? At the end of each day of observation in the French nursing home, I relayed my hesitations in the notes that I took in my car, in the parking lot of the facility. I tried to reflect on my hesitations in the frame of this system of deference production that I was both analyzing and navigating in. Displaying this uncertainty will, I hope, enable us to ascertain that taking some distance from the humanist discourse does not reduce the merit of the professionals who work hard to enact its values; on the contrary, this aims at insisting on this complex series of microdecisions and actions that cannot simply be accounted for as values.[9]

> November 22: I have a better understanding of the difficulties of care this afternoon. It was the weekly bingo game that took place in the main room [there are both residents diagnosed with dementia and suffering from various disabilities]. While I help Marie-Pierre [who is in charge of entertainment] to install the tables, a resident, Mrs. Fromentin, calls me. "Sir, I hardly see anything anymore. Usually there's someone who stands beside me and helps me." She is afraid that no one will help her. I take this opportunity to find myself a place. I propose to Marie-Pierre that I will "take care" of this table. It is a circular table where three residents are seated. In front of me, Mrs. Fromentin, who cannot stand the brightness of the room. Eye problems. She wears big sunglasses and asks me to sit in such a way as to hide the light of a lamp behind me. I am therefore positioned in a most precise way. She seems to hear rather well and to have the ability to concentrate. On my left, Mrs. Glacis, a resident whom I find quite complicated to understand. I have already met her several times, as she was walking around in the main room, using a tripod cane. She then used to give me a big smile and kept waving to say "hi," probably. She has some difficulty articulating (so I do not know

whether it is a diction problem or if she just says anything). At the table, she continues to smile at me blissfully. Finally, to my right, a rather shadowy resident, Mrs. Patouilleaux, huddled on her bingo grid, who hardly hears anything despite her hearing device and deliberately sulks. She seems to see correctly and does not have any cognitive impairment.

I find myself in the position of a goodwill beginner: I use all the visible signs in the residents' behavior in order to estimate their capacities, in order to know how to give them some help during the bingo game, which, let us not forget, is taken very seriously. That the game begins three minutes late arouses some irritation among the residents, who also do not like that Marie-Pierre takes the opportunity when announcing the numbers to make jokes. Bingo is serious. For my part, I wish to show my ability to contribute to the nursing home life, feeling that I am still considered a Parisian bookish type dropped here by the director.

The game begins. Focus is at its height among the forty residents participating. Each time Marie-Pierre announces a number, I try to estimate whether the residents of my table have heard the number [hearing impairment compensation] and check whether they have put a pawn on their grid in case they have the right number [visual and possibly cognitive impairment compensation].

I experience a first surprise while Marie-Pierre announces the third number. Mrs. Glacis recognizes a number on her grid and puts a pawn on it. Seeing this, Mrs. Patouilleaux exclaims, "What? The game started?" I had forgotten to warn her, failing to anticipate that she would not hear at all. From that moment, I systematically repeat the numbers announced by Marie-Pierre, to be sure that Mrs. Patouilleaux hears. I'm not comfortable, and, I think, neither is the resident. I realize why after five minutes. Repeating the numbers certainly allows her not to miss anything, but it displays her hearing problems, loudly, in a group structured primarily by the visibility of impairment marks [the residents form friendly groups organized by degree of visible handicap. The most able groups, such as Mrs. Patouilleaux's friends, reject and make fun of the less able. Residents visibly suffering from dementia are sidelined and arouse embarrassed silences when they walk into common rooms]. By repeating the numbers systematically, I may make her difficulties public, threatening her sociability. I stop routinely repeating the numbers and regularly look inquiringly to the resident to know if I have to repeat.

Another difficulty arises when I try to help Mrs. Fromentin. She leans so that her eyes are about ten centimeters from her grid. Every time Marie-Pierre announces a number, I check that she does not miss it on her grid. When she misses it, it seems difficult to tell her without sounding infantilizing. I have to speak loudly. The resident hears decently enough but only to a certain extent. Therefore I have to graduate my indications to help her the least amount possible whilst trying not to appear too infantilizing, whilst also being quite helpful. "You have it," I was saying at first. "More up/left/right/down," I was saying if she did not get it. Then I pointed to the number on the grid. She used to say "thanks" but in a grumbling tone.

When residents mistake a number, I tell them, but it's hard not to look contemptuous. To speak overpolitely and cautiously seems to be the best way. According to my standards, to note an error without raising the associated impairment is best: "excuse me, but I think you have mistaken the number. I think it is not the right one." First of all, to speak in a way that is consistent with the written regulations suggests that I need to emphasize the "respect" due to the elderly persons. And I realize that I reproduce the same behavioral traits that I observed among health professionals in cases of discreditation. . . . I notice that Marie-Pierre dissipates this discomfort by another technique: teasing. "So Mrs. Germain, are we getting muddled up?" I find that it is quite friendly, less infantilizing than my method, but I do not know the residents well enough to do it. . . .

Finally, with Mrs. Glacis, I realize gradually that she is not losing her mind at all, and I wonder if I should keep checking her grid. She realizes that I look at her grid when each number is announced and gives me the same smile every time. After a few minutes, however, I realize that she is never wrong. But I take some time to double check before I stop. Monitoring the grid: not excluding someone from the game. At the same time, this line of action is potentially infantilizing. Dilemma. Twice, I repeat the number to her, and she tells me that she already knew it. It is also possible that she "makes up for it" to save face.

I think that many things play out in the efforts made to find a "fair" voice tone and posture—that is to say, which are perceived by the interlocutor as expressing some kindness without making them feel infantilized. I mostly struggle to place my voice. It is actually difficult to speak loudly without giving this infantilizing impression. With some residents, you have to touch them and look at them very closely to catch their attention. Without giving the impression of talking to a child . . .

[The following week, I am "promoted," and I now announce the bingo numbers myself] I announce the first numbers, and I realize that I did not say them loud enough. Half of the residents did not even notice that the game had started. . . . I increase the volume of my voice for the following numbers, but my tone seems very dry, almost irritated. It sounds like I'm not happy to be here. I try to soften it by making it more "tonal," but it sounds very quickly infantilizing. I think I find the "right" after fifteen minutes. But how to describe it?

My difficulties partly stemmed from my personal situation, for I have never had to take care of an elderly person, and my posture as a sociologist, which consists of questioning everything, including my own behavior. Nonetheless, I found the same difficulties in the stories staff members related to me. While managers told me that the relational aspect of work has been widely developed in nursing aides' training, nursing aides themselves often report that they were not prepared by their training for the situations encountered. For example, they are trained to perform technical gestures such as waking residents up and making them eat and go to bed. In being trained to perform these gestures, nursing aides practice with their colleagues, taking them as "guinea pigs" who are, of course, rather docile. Once they start working in institutions, they find themselves faced with residents who may not be compliant and must then relearn "on the job" to act in such a way as to generate docility. In sum, producing deference "appropriately" toward the elderly, especially those suffering from cognitive trouble, is a social learned skill.

To develop this point, staff members told me what inspired them when they started working with people suffering from cognitive impairments. Some evoked a previous experience in their personal lives, such as having taken care of an elderly relative or a child; through these experiences, to take Stacey's words, they acquired an "emotional capital" usable in their work.[10] These experiences prepare them for the attentive, patient, and caring attitude necessary for their current work. Others explain that they derive these skills from their "culture" of origin, as this nursing aide, a native of Morocco, said:

> In our country, nursing homes are very rare. It's new to me . . . but helping people, helping people, being available for them, doing whatever they want doesn't cause me any problems. . . . But we don't have nursing homes or shelters in Morocco. . . . There you take care of your mother or grandmother until their death. Even . . . for example, you

may take care of your mother-in-law too. You can ... you may under-take part-time work. ... You may make sacrifices to help them, even leave your job. Even a neighbor, you may take care of her! So, the tasks, yes, I'm used to them.

Some staff members recounted past work experiences, whether in the care and education sectors or in the service sector. A former nightclub worker drew similarities with his previous job: "When you're a waiter, and you serve a drink, if you pull a face, nobody will like the drink. It's the same thing here. If you pull a face, the resident won't want it. There's not only the drink, there's the service that goes with it." In addition to previous experiences and train-ings, the emotional and technical assistance received from col-leagues is significant.[11] Colleagues exchange "tricks" and suggest helpful ways of proceeding and generally support each other.

Some common relational techniques emerge from these mixed influences, even if they are almost never formalized in this way. The employees, both in France and in Quebec, maintain the sense that they do instinctive rather than overly technical work. They do not consider the reflexes acquired on the job expertise as such. That said, we can discern five different relation techniques, to which I now turn.

First, *nonverbal deduction*, which is introduced well by Tarik, a nursing aide I met during the research: "With the elderly who don't have any cognitive trouble, if they're hungry they ask, if they are thirsty they ask, if they want something they ask. But with Al-zheimer's we must guess. We must go by deduction. We give drinks, food, and after a while we find what the matter is." In order to de-duce the expectations of the residents, three sources of clues are essential: the look (a sad or joyful expression, the direction of the eyes), facial expressions (smile, frown), and "small sounds" (types of moaning, words). The ability to recognize these signs increases as the nursing aide gets to know the resident.

Second, *emotional work* is a concept developed by Arlie Hoch-schild[12] as a means to designate the work done on oneself to give the impression that one experiences the emotions appropriate to a given situation. Employees, nurses, and nursing aides undertake emotional work in order to experience effectively appropriate emotions and to communicate the same type of emotions to their interlocutors. This sort of emotional work was mentioned regularly in many of the interviews. Employees explained that they have to face a very wide range of affects[13] and have to make sure they are in a good mood at work, to "last" their shift. With residents who no longer communicate with words, a "positive" state of mind helps to encourage cooperation. Lydia explained: "The emotions, they feel them. If you arrive in the morning and you're in a bad mood, you're going to have trouble approaching them. They do not know why, but they feel it." Since staff members are in constant contact with ill, elderly people who are likely to die in the near future, they must also control their own affects, especially when they return home. This problem seems to vary according to seniority in the profession, as the oldest staff members reported this type of problem less while the new ones spoke of it abundantly and were reassured in the workplace by the oldest employees. Nadia, who had been working for six months as a nursing aide, said that she found it hard to sleep and to stop thinking about residents when she returned home. "But they [my colleagues] told me that with time I won't stay like that. They said, 'You're going to get used to it'. . . . They say, 'it did that to us as well, at the beginning, it's a passage we all pass through.'"

Third, the *setting up of daily rituals* occupies a large part of the time of the nursing aides, since their work mainly concerns repetitive situations that occur every day, such as taking meals, waking up, showering, and so on. Nursing aides learn the different habits of each resident as they go along. Nathalie gives us an idea of what is at stake: "Place the table at such an angle, not too much at the right, not too much at the left, put the phone there, the glass on the left, the straw at the right. . . . It's a lot of little stuff like that. Putting the cover on the shoulders, or on the neck. . . . They each have their own little habits. If you don't know them, the resident loses patience." Although employees generally describe these gestures as "little tricks" or "small things," their fulfilment contributes significantly to the satisfaction expressed by the residents or their relatives. Moreover, attention to the "little things" also enables employees to keep pace with the increasing rhythm of work due to budget cuts. "When you have five minutes [per patient] you need to know. If you don't know it can take up to thirty minutes," Joel summarized.

Fourth, the *use of the residents' past* requires having previously gathered information about this past through the family, other professionals, or the patients when they still can express themselves. This information is useful because it provides topics for conversation with nonspeaking residents, which allows for more individualized interaction than small talk about the weather, for instance. It is also useful to be familiar with the patient's past when staff are required to interpret behaviors that do not make sense at first sight. The final "function" of knowing the past is that it provides opportunities for staff to "make diversions," a very important element in the work of nursing aides. By evoking a memory, such as an old occupation, a nursing aide can change the focus and even the ideas of a resident while eating or taking a shower, thus facilitating the ease of their tasks. This will be addressed in greater detail in the next chapter.

The fifth and final technique is the *creation, or production, of interaction rites*. When we "know" someone, creating interaction rites can manifest as certain rituals that are unique to this relationship, oftentimes in the form of "private jokes." These rites construct the relation; they individualize the relation in the sense that they make it different from all the others. If this type of activity is common to all social relations, nursing aides practice it in a singular way, since their interlocutors can have weakened cognitive abilities. Xavier took the example of a nonspeaking resident that greeted him with a military salute. "It makes her laugh! She likes me!" he commented. Paul evoked his jokes concerning the surname of a resident. "Mrs. Thanh Thai, listen, her name is Mrs. Thanh Thai, but I never call her like that. Well, when her family comes in, I call her Mrs. Thanh Thai, but otherwise I call her Ms. Ping Ping. I don't know how, it came to me like that. When I see her it's 'hello, Ms. Ping Ping, how are you?' . . . then she's all happy." Similar to the interactions in which the staff members make use of the residents' past, these created rites serve to distract residents and build rapport with those who cannot communicate.

We must, however, keep the backstage in mind. First, increasing work rhythms give employees less time to develop their interaction skills and their "relational style" in more depth.[14] Second, the representation conveyed by the media and official job descriptions distinguishes between clearly identified physical tasks (washing patients, helping them to wake up, etc.) *and* the relational aspect, which is often presented in vague and moralistic terms. Here is the job description of a nursing aide displayed on *Avenir en Santé*, a website managed by the Quebec Ministry of Health and Social Services: "Orderlies help patients in the morning, during meals, and at bedtime. They help them bathe, dress or undress, and are responsible for the bedding. They provide patients with the appropriate care and respect their integrity and dignity with an aim towards contributing to their well-being."

Again, the deference required presents as a set of values, as if it were a given moral attitude that one would have to possess. On the contrary, we have seen that producing deference, knowing how to behave with patients, especially when they suffer from cognitive impairments, and dealing with the complex situations arising from it can be, or rather must be, learned. Nobody is ever really "sure" of the outcome. What is more, failing to recognize the relational work of employees (in the nursing home sector as well as in the home assistance sector) as a competence amounts to the imposition of responsibility for which they are not explicitly trained. Placing emphasis on their moral attitude diverts questioning about the organization of work, its rhythm, the training provided, and the abstract nature of the values to be followed. That is to say, the social conditions that shape their professional activity are invisibilized.

Neither Hospitals nor Hotels: Nursing Homes as "Secondary Institutions"

In any institution, there are standards of deference governing the relationships between the different groups that interact together. I will distinguish here *primary institutions*, in which these relations are self-referenced, from *secondary institutions*, in which these re-lations tend to follow the models of other institutions.[15]

A quick comparison will help to clarify these notions. Schools are primary institutions where the relationship between teachers and pupils, in particular, acts as a reference model as such. The typical remarks of some teachers suggest that school is in itself a model to follow when they remind their pupils that they are "not in a circus" if the students are unruly or "at home" when their outfits do not meet the standards of the institution. Or even when students do not want their school to resemble a "prison" if teachers are too authoritarian and when some opponents to the increasing privatization of schools claim that education sector "is not a su-permarket" nor "a company." I do not think I am mistaken in as-suming that school as an institution makes sense to most people, that there is an imagination of what the teacher/pupil relationship is or should be, and that this ideal model is widely accepted. When stakeholders aim to change these relations, it is to establish a better model of teacher/pupil relationship and nothing else.

Nursing homes are, on the contrary, secondary institutions. For professionals as well as for residents and their families, the worst that can happen to these facilities is that they resemble . . . nursing homes. When I arrived at one of these facilities in Quebec to meet with a manager, she started by highlighting this aspect. At the entrance of the building was a fireplace, much decorated walls, some "vintage" armchairs, and a janitor who made jokes to the passers-by.

THE MANAGER: You see that the atmosphere is special?

Yes. When I arrived, I met Eric [the janitor], and there are chairs, it's warm, and it does not seem . . .

THE MANAGER: Like a nursing home? [Proud] Yes, it's special!

While the administrative and architectural structures of the facilities are often those of hospitals (sometimes because they are old hospitals converted), the model of the hospital constitutes the ultimate repellent. The "change of culture" in the housing sector for the elderly has, in fact, led to a disqualification of the hospital and the associated traditional models (hospice) in favor of other models: the *hotel* and the *home*. Quite often, when the actors of an institution "in crisis" want to change its brand image, they try to make it resemble institutions carrying more positive connotations, as when some parishes intend to "rejuvenate" their images by decorating the catechism rooms as youth cultural centers.

I discussed this process widely with the director of the institution where I conducted my observations in France. This private facility belongs to one of the largest companies in the sector. Its building was constructed a few years ago. The architecture is modern and includes attractive facilities such as a balneotherapy room and a multisensory space. Significantly, this is the only institution where my request to conduct fieldwork was accepted, out of twenty requests. At a period of time during which the media repeatedly focused on scandals regarding abuse of residents, this acceptance required the agreement of the *communication* department of the head office. This facility appears to be a showcase for the company, which suggests that the director's narrative is in line with the current strategies of the sector.

For the director, the challenge is to move from the model of the hospital to the hotel. In other words, residents should not feel as if they are the patients of a health structure but the guests of a pleasant inn. We find here the question of deference again, since what matters in this shift is the status that residents must have (as guests) and the feeling of belonging through the relationships forged with professionals. To effect this change from hospital to hotel, the director said that he kept this distinction in mind at every stage during the planning of the new building. The colors of the walls, for example, were carefully chosen in order to differentiate themselves from hospital colors. Beige has been preferred to white and warm colors instead of pastel colors. Residents are encouraged to decorate the doors of their rooms and hang their photographs so that when they walk the corridors, they and their visitors do not feel as though they are meandering monotonously through a hospital. Professionals use vaporizers to hide the often unpleasant smell that prevails in these places. Cleaning products typically used in house-holds are also selected in favor of industrial bleach, for instance, the odor of which is often associated with hospitals. Managers limit the use of mobile nursing carts, which characterize hospitals, not least because of the wheel noises on the ground. The height of the electric plugs provoked some debates. The director wanted them to be close to the ground, as in any home or hotel, unlike hospitals and "ordinary" nursing homes (where they are located forty inches from the ground to easily connect to medical devices). But they were finally placed at forty inches for fear that placing the power points any lower would incur legal ramifications. That is to say, the legal framework relevant to the institution remains that of a hospital, with the safety standards of a hospital, more constraining than those of a hotel.

In Quebec, where I have focused on the public sector, the managers interviewed expressed the same rejection of the hospital model but instead gave priority to the "living environment" or "home" model—the units are called, literally, "life units" (*unités de vie*). This means that residents must feel at home in a family-like atmosphere. Such an orientation also results in policies that regulate decorations. Several recommendations of the minister, for example, require that facilities do not look like hospitals: "the administrative display is eliminated in the units"; "the display above the resident's beds is eliminated [with some exceptions]"; "no bed-linen is placed on the beds or at the doors of the rooms before the bedtime of the residents." Employees are discouraged from wearing overly formal attire, in order to privilege clothing that resembles "everyday life." Also, it is recommended that all residents be permitted variable bedtimes, because in a "life environment," everyone sleeps when they want. The home model implies a greater personalization of services, as this executive suggested:

> In the nursing home we try to make it look like a living environment so that it is as most personalized as possible. So, you dress with your clothes, your room is with your taste . . . so your room should not look like that of the neighbor, because it's like your house, or your apartment. It doesn't resemble that of the neighbor because it's your

personality. There's what you love in there. Then, for example, the meal. How am I positioned? Do I have good eye contact? Do I name what I am serving? A lot happens in the relationship and how the staff are acting.

This line of action strongly impacts the organization of work. For the workers that I met, creating a living environment amounts to disrupting the traditional division of institutional work. Each professional has a set of defined tasks and sticks to it in order to set up a less rigid organization in which each professional has a set of tasks but must adapt depending on the needs of the residents. An oft cited example is maintenance workers, who have to "give a hand" if they see a resident in trouble or another employee overworked. Finally, the changes in managerial logics underway approximate those of other workplaces, which are becoming more "flexible." This flexibility can be observed in *start-ups* with the supposed informality of their employees' attitude.

In one of the observed facilities, a manager thus presented its organization in "scattered tasks":

The specificity here, it's the "scattered tasks." By "scattered tasks" I mean that . . . at lunch, you have an employee who makes the toast. It won't prevent the nursing assistant and nursing aide from giving a hand. José, who is on the housekeeping, he can very well make some intervention to prepare residents, to take residents to the dining room or to mass. At 10:00 a.m., there is a nursing aide who arrives and stays until 6:00 p.m. Her main task will be the organization of lunch and dinner. She takes care of the kitchen, and she puts the plates on the bar while another employee serves. *There's no nursing aide who passes by with a cart; it's not a hospital.* When deliveries [of food] arrive, it is this aide who takes deliveries, puts fresh produce in the fridge, arranges things, and takes them out for the meal. Elsewhere, the food department delivers everything already prepared. So this nursing aide has an important position.

As can be gleaned from these transcripts, we can note a further distinction between those nursing homes that seek to avoid any association with "the hospital," those that embrace the image of "the hotel," and those that embrace that of "the home." The difference between the institutions oriented toward the model of the home and those that follow the model of the hotel can be observed through a few details. Because they said they felt too passive, some residents of the French facility asked to help with the preparation of meals, by offering to peel vegetables or set the table. They were refused the opportunity: "They are here to rest," claimed an entertainment coordinator when I spoke to her. Which hotel restaurant would accept that guests would prepare their own meals? However, negotiations sometimes take place between professionals and those residents deemed most able, who want to clean their own rooms. They may be allowed to do so and, even if not, may do the housekeeping themselves before an employee arrives to do it. In the facilities observed in Quebec, some residents were allowed to participate in domestic tasks. "We let her fold the tea towels and aprons. She likes it very much," a manager commented. In a living environment, everyone is invited to participate. All the residents endorse the refusal of the hospital and the nursing home models. They do so by manifesting their desire to distance themselves, as much as possible, from these despised models and the attributes that symbolize them. In the French facility, such a distancing appeared in the refusal to wear one's "emergency call button." This was particularly significant, as the button is worn around the neck, visibly differentiating residents who wear it or not. Further, there is a collective reluctance to name the wheelchairs "wheelchairs," privileging other expressions such as "small car," "this stuff," "the machine," and "the wheeled machine."

Despite these attempts at differentiating the facilities from the model of the hospital, employees tend to keep the hospital model as a reference—in both a negative and a positive sense. Those who previously worked in general hospital services say that they no longer spend their days pursuing medical tasks and instead focus on something "human." They describe their career orientation as a transition from the medical world to the psychological world. Those who were working outside the health or care sector also consider their move as oriented toward a medical sector where patients are looked after. This persistence of the hospital model is partly linked to the administrative structure of their employment, largely modeled on the scales, organizational schemes, and division of work at play in the hospital sector.

Conclusion

From the moment someone is suspected of suffering from dementia, the deference to which they are subject progressively becomes a moral then an organizational stake. People around them tend to question the "best" way of behaving toward them. The health services supporting those suspected of suffering from dementia partly structure their own interventions with these patients around the institutional production of deference. The social experience of dementia—through the interactions to which patients have access—is thus structured by those (mainly institutional) issues.

Deference production takes place through antagonistic movements. Most nursing home professionals try to ensure that their facility does not look like a nursing home, let alone a hospital—in a way that ill residents feel, as little as possible, that they are ill and residents. They do so despite acting within the administrative and legal framework of a hospital structure, with a hierarchy of professions and tasks based on the hospital model, with the same priority accorded to safety, and so forth.[16] Another antagonism is that the tendency to frame the deference as preferably "spontaneous," drawing on "authentic" moral attitudes,[17] occurs alongside the multiplication of means of control and planning and the increasing rhythms of work. The home care sector follows the same path, valuing the "human" while building an "arsenal of regulatory devices and standard procedures," which Bernard Ennuyer (about the French case, but this applies in most Western countries) regrets takes precedence over ethical issues.[18]

How can we understand this *bureaucratization of humanism*? First, I wish to note that this process mostly follows the prophetic observations of Max Weber[19] regarding the increasing dominance of bureaucratic forms of organization over Western societies. Furthermore, in the history of care institutions for the elderly, we observe a process similar to that which Luc Boltanski and Eve Chiapello[20] observed in the world of work in general. The social movements of the 1960s, those encouraging self-management, individual freedom, creativity, and less institutional confinement, were taken over by management consultants and company executives. The latter have reformulated principles pointing toward a critique *of* companies as a tool for change *in* companies. Hence the new labor organizations where employees, supposedly flexible and autonomous, "would benefit from the advice" of their manager instead of "obeying orders" from their boss. The same story can be read off of health-care institutions. It would be easy to see that the critical movements regarding these institutions, especially in the 1950s, 1960s, and 1970s, which denounced a lack of "humanity" in the care of patients and the elderly, have been integrated into organizations: *humanist criticism has become a management tool.*

This movement has permitted a more systematic production of deference, which is likely more in line with collective morality. The "quality of services," to take a local expression, seems to have improved overall, at least in comparison with the hospices of yesteryear. But it is not that simple. We are currently at a pivotal moment when the deference produced tends to become institutionalized in the form of standardized grids of "good" and "bad" behaviors. A moment when the humanist approach to care engenders a stereotyped mode of interaction whereby, instead of integrating one's interlocutors into "common humanity" by behaving with them as with others, these interlocutors are in fact differentiated from others, as they are offered a set of behaviors specific to all those who share the same diagnosis, receive the same services, or live in the same institution. A moment when professionals, often overwhelmed, do not have any more margin to reflect on this topic and can only save time by following the guidelines that are supposed to ensure the realization of their own values.

4

RECONSTITUTING PEOPLE

THIS AFTERNOON, A PHOTOGRAPHY ACTIVITY IS PLANNED WITH a professional photographer who is equipped with a mobile studio. The activity director hopes to mobilize families, who have the opportunity to take some nice pictures with their relatives, the subtext being the creation of a beautiful memory, perhaps the last one. The mobile studio is set at 2:00 p.m., and Mrs. Sinclair arrives first in a wheelchair pushed by her daughter. She does not react to what is being said to her. She seems to live in "another world." Her head leaning to one side and with a tottering look, she wears pink slippers, sweatpants, and a blue T-shirt with a pink vest. She does not speak, sometimes emitting a few barely audible groans.

Mrs. Sinclair is greeted by the photographer, who addresses her as if she were a child, using a very contrived voice. The photographer accompanies her words with sweeping gestures and addresses Mrs. Sinclair in the third person. The activity director, the daughter, and photographer interact with Ms. Sinclair in front of a small crowd of residents who make some occasional comments. A photography workshop, what a great opportunity for gossip! I remain silent.

PHOTOGRAPHER: Want to take a photo?

ACTIVITY DIRECTOR: Yes, you will let her take some pictures of you, right, Mrs. Sinclair?

DAUGHTER: Come on, let's go!

The activity director calls a staff member to help her move Mrs. Sinclair from her wheelchair to the decorated chair. The session begins. While the photographer takes a few shots while "conversing" with the resident, the daughter explains that her mother used to have a photography studio with her deceased spouse. She hopes this environment may help her mother recall a few things, or at the very least cause some sort of reaction, however small. A few moments later, Mrs. Sinclair slightly contracts her cheeks, mostly the left one, unveiling some teeth. The activity director exclaims, "Well, you see! She recalls something! Hey, Mrs. Sinclair, it looks familiar to you, doesn't it?" The director then turns to the photographer, who did not understand. "She used to work in a photography shop!"

This new information seems to help the photographer significantly, as she appeared to have exhausted all conversational possibilities with her model. "So you worked in a photography studio? With your husband?" The daughter answers: "Yes, with my father." The photographer then shows the cameras to the resident, giving some technical details. The activity director comments, "You would have seen a lot of cameras like that, huh?"

After a while, the photographer wants to spice up the shoot. She has brought hats of multiple shapes and colors. She chooses the soberer one, a black hat, a choice maybe impelled by the resident's inability to speak. Would putting the pink one on—as the resident cannot express any consent—have been inappropriate? Anyway, the hat seems to make Mrs. Sinclair "smile" a little more. This causes another wave of enthusiasm. "She smiles! She likes it!" exclaims the activity director. The daughter nods. The photographer tries to sustain the smile of the resident: "It looks good on you. You are beautiful with this hat. . . . I'm gonna take great pictures, you'll see. You'll be very, very surprised!"

After a few shots, the photographer takes Mrs. Sinclair's hand and positions her elbow on the armrest of the chair so that her hand touches the hat. It seems as though the activity director is attempting to recreate a Michael Jackson-like pose. Everyone laughs again in response to the "smile" of the resident that only slightly expands. Mrs. Sinclair then receives a lot of compliments until the end of the photo shoot session.

The last phase of the shooting consists of reviewing the pictures on the photographer's laptop. I feel that the interlocutors are short of ideas to sustain the "conversation," hence the repetitive character of the notes that I take at the moment: "You see, you are beautiful!"; "That hat suits you well!"; "The hat shows you off"; "You're very beautiful like that"; "Your photos are great, Mrs. Sinclair!", and so on.

Filling the Gaps in the Present Interaction: Reconstitution Work

During the exchanges I have just described, it should be noted that the people around Mrs. Sinclair struggled to maintain any interaction with her, since she did not speak and her facial expressions were difficult to interpret. In order to be able to interact, the photographer, the activity director, and the daughter *reconstituted* what would have happened *if* the resident were not ill and thereby simulated interactions with her by asking her questions as if she were going to answer, then imagining her answers.

The fact that people with dementia, at some stage of the disease, are no longer able to communicate in the usual way gives rise to a type of activity that I call *reconstitution*. Reconstitution involves introducing into an interaction some elements designed to simulate what the persons would do or say if they could interact "normally"; note that this notion is close to the notion of "assisted self-presentation," coined by Næss et al. in the same setting.[1]

Nursing home staff members regularly resort to this type of interaction—for example, at mealtimes. They must seek the consent of residents to feed them while residents may not always be able to express consent, whether they are hungry, and what they like to eat or not. Faced with the dilemma, the employees simulate this consent:

Hello, Ms. Smith, are you feeling well today?
[Silence]

You want to eat? Are you hungry?
[Silence]
Very good! Today we have mixed chicken. Is it okay with you?
[Silence]
That's good, isn't it?
[Silence]

In nursing home units welcoming residents diagnosed with dementia at an advanced stage, reconstitution activities become a common form of communication. Interacting with people who are almost or wholly incomprehensible then requires a disposition to improvisation:

> [I am in the office of a manager, whom I observe working by taking notes, Quebec] 13:25. A woman enters the room, the door of which was open. She groans and drools. Emilie, the manager, does not pay attention. She slightly raises her eyebrows when the resident goes out, apparently to see if I am uneasy. 13.30. The woman returns. She wails and emits low groans, a little anxious, I guess. Head aside. Stands in front of Emilie's office and continues to groan. Emilie, after a moment, mimics some surprise, as if the resident had just told her something: "Yes?" She sighs. "Have you eaten well today?" The resident makes turns and looks at me. Emilie, very gently (like to a child): "Well, yes, I have a visitor today." The resident goes out. Emilie comments, "This lady comes every day. She's been here for five years. It's an Alzheimer's disease, a kind of rapid dementia, something like that. . . . Sometimes she comes and she's there. We can talk to her about everyday things like "it's cold" or what I ate, but sometimes it happens that there is no one upstairs [meaning in her mind]. You can see that the eyes, there's nothing, she's no longer here. But in general you can talk to her as for a daily conversation."

The reconstitution work may also take a collective twist when, in Alzheimer units, employees seek to create a more "lively" atmosphere. In one of these units, the daily life seems immutable. Twelve residents sit around a large square table. Nobody moves or speaks. Only a few groans or disorganized gestures occasionally break the background noise radiated by the television. The two professionals who are in charge of the unit that day, Steven and Adama, are speaking to one another, though within earshot of the residents. They are never certain that they are understood or even heard. Both fans of soccer, they talk about yesterday's game and "exchange" their impressions with random residents, knowing that none of them will probably ever answer.

ADAMA: Didier Deschamps [the captain of the French national team], everything he does, he succeeds. Trust me, we're on the right path there. . . . We're on the good track!

STEVEN [SMILING]: You saw yesterday. . . .

ADAMA: They played . . . as they did in '98! [When France won the World Cup]

[Silence]

ADAMA: So, France at the World Cup, what d'you think of that, Mrs. Dunod? [No answer] And Mr. Gomez, d'you prefer Italy or Germany? [No answer]

STEVEN: Eh! He goes for Spain! Mr. Gomez! It's for Spain!

[Silence]

ADAMA [TO ME AND HIS COLLEAGUE]: Me, I tell you, Didier Deschamps, everything he does, he succeeds!

Some of this collective reconstitution work is more planned, becoming an institutional device, as I observed during the weekly bingo game in France. Among the forty usual participants, a table was reserved for those who could not play because they were either too cognitively impaired or too sleepy, or indeed some combination of both. An employee then had to make the residents play, often because their family had asked them to or because they used to play when they were able to. When a number is announced, the employee went around the table, checked the grids of each player, and, slaloming between the wheelchairs, played each grid by putting pawns on the relevant square when required. The whole bingo game lasted one hour and a half.

Reconstitution can also consist of inventing narrative elements in order to build jokes—reconstituting, then, what could be but is not.

> Asma visits her colleagues in a different unit than the one she is in charge of. She points to an immobile resident in a chair: "Eh, you take good care of my mother-in-law, eh!"
> Farid, her colleague, exclaims, "Yes, it's like your mother-in-law is a in four-star hotel!" [Laughs]

> Asma: "Oh, yes, because you have to be careful, I tell you, to my mother-in-law, or you'll get a clip around the ear!" [Some residents look; some seem amused; others seem not to understand]
> Farid: "When did you get married to her son, then?"
> Asma: "Robert? Oh! Very soon!"
> A resident rushes to Asma: "Are you going to get married, young woman?"
> Asma: "Yes, soon, Mrs. Pierre, when the weather is fine."
> Resident: "Oh, so you're up the creek without a paddle!"

Employees use this behavior both for the purpose of "winding down" in emotionally stressful work situations and for animating those units where the residents do not speak, with the exception of the occasional moan. However, reconstitutions made for joking may be frowned upon by executives, other employees, or the relatives of the residents should they be interpreted as "disrespect." It is not because the residents cannot react that we must allow ourselves to tell them anything, they say. The managers of Asma, for example, seriously remonstrated with her in the days that followed the reported jesting. Mostly anticipating the possible reactions from visiting families, they considered her humor inappropriate.

But for employees, those reconstitutions aimed at making jokes have some utility. They provide them with an opportunity to react to the destabilizing behaviors of some residents. Indeed, as many of their interlocutors suffer from severe cognitive disorders, the interactions may take an epic dimension. In addition, since most residents lose their memories in the short term, all that is said can be forgotten five minutes later: the exchanges are above all meant to fill the present moment. The information exchanged becomes less "serious" than usual; it engages only the here and now. Residents are often disoriented, do not realize where they are, or imagine being elsewhere, doing something else, and so on. Since it is admitted that staff members should consequently better focus on the present than to continuously reframe residents, they develop a behavioral repertoire intending to turn a strange routine into some potentially funny interactions. In particular, this process can be observed when residents ask for the same thing on several occasions:

> A resident, Mrs. Vallée, approaches an employee, Sandrine, pointing to me: Who is this young man?
>
> Sandrine, articulating: It is Baptiste Brossard. He comes to see how things happen here.
>
> Mrs. Vallée, suspicious: Ah. [She leaves]
>
> [Five minutes later]
>
> Mrs. Vallée approaches Sandrine, pointing to me: Who is this young man?
>
> Sandrine: It's Baptiste. He comes to see how it goes on here.
>
> Mrs. Vallée, suspicious: Ah. [She leaves]
>
> [Five minutes later]
>
> Mrs. Vallée approaches Sandrine, pointing to me: Who is this young man?
>
> Sandrine: It's Baptiste, he's . . . [sighs] . . . he's a researcher. A sociologist.
>
> Mrs. Vallée, suspicious: Ah. [She leaves]
>
> [Five minutes later]
>
> Mrs. Vallée approaches Sandrine, pointing to me: Who is this young man?
>
> Sandrine (laughing): Baptiste. That's my friend!
>
> Mrs. Vallée, suspicious: Ah. [She leaves]
>
> [fie minutes later]
>
> Mrs. Vallée approaches Sandrine, pointing to me: Who is this young man?
>
> Sandrine (exclaims nervously, eyes wide open): It's Baptiste. It's my son!
>
> Mrs. Vallée, surprised: Ah? Nice to meet you, Baptiste!

Travelling in Time: The Social Content of Reconstitution

Since it is impossible to know anyone perfectly, we must always rely on reconstructions. In the manner of detectives, we use clues about the past of our interlocutors (what they did, the tastes they expressed, the behaviors they had) in order to reconstruct their "personality" through a series of hypotheses (so-and-so has had such behavior, so they have such a type of personality). We introduce this hypothetical knowledge in our exchanges with our interlocutors. The gift is a ritualized form of this work of reconstruction. When you give a gift to someone, you reflect on what you know about that person to imagine what you can offer. Your gift thus demonstrates your knowledge of this person who, in return, might express joy in the face of this gift, in part because it displays a mutual knowledge. Studies regarding this ritual show that social stereotypes are used widely when offering gifts, especially when one is unfamiliar with the recipient and when the gift giver has few "clues" from the past of the recipient. For example, women are more likely to be offered cooking utensils while men are more generally offered alcohol, thereby reproducing traditions in gender, class, and age relationships.[2]

With people at an advanced stage of dementia who are unable to communicate in a conventional manner, this reconstruction work occurs on an unprecedented scale. Interactions rely explicitly and exclusively on reconstitution, simply because it is the only possible option. Moreover, the diagnosed elderly progressively cease to provide the people surrounding them with new clues, partly because it is increasingly considered that their behavior is expressive of their disease and not their "personality" (recalling the process of discreditation). Hence the emergence of a belief that holds that the "true self" of those diagnosed is no longer "here" and the elements of the past are more "authentic" than those of the present.

Consequently, in order to interact with the patients, to show them some deference, their interlocutors undertake reconstitutions based on their belonging to various social groups. I list below three possible strategies by which interlocutors undertake such processes of reconstitution:

First, dementia patients can be associated with the "*normals.*" I borrow this expression from Sue Estroff, whose study of psychiatric outpatients shows that these patients think of themselves as "crazy" in opposition to "normal."[3] A set of behaviors constitutes interlocutors' attempts to associate those suffering from dementia with the imaginary group of supposedly normal people. In particular, greeting rituals thus highlight that receivers, as "normal" people, deserve to be greeted with "sir," "madame," "good morning," or "how are you?" The patients' interlocutors seem to insist on these formulas, stressing that if patients are in specific situations or even live in institutions, they benefit from the same considerations as anyone. This is probably one of the reasons why greeting rituals are much more pronounced in nursing homes than in non-institutional environments. Employees say "hello" separately and insistently, followed by the person's name. Most importantly, such greetings are deployed even, or especially, in cases when it is unclear whether the recipient of the greeting can hear or understand it at all. The same process can be observed with home help professionals.

Consider another example: some jokes consist of simulating a conversation as if the patient were young and/or proceed as if the affected individual were not so affected. For instance, when a nursing home resident asks a caregiver to arrange an outing to the market, the caregiver responds, "You want to meet a handsome young man, right?" In another instance, a nursing aide addresses a visibly disoriented resident in the corridor of a facility: "Are you going to the ball, Mr. Lafitte?" Through this set of rites, a form of "normality," or at least an escape from the restrictions related to the disease, is staged.

Second, some behaviors enacted when conversing with dementia patients suggest that their recipient belongs to a *specific group*. People diagnosed with dementia are mostly considered members of "the elderly" group. Often, professionals and the family circle produce signs of consideration focused on the age of the patient. The "reminiscence spaces," currently very fashionable in nursing homes, probably constitute the apotheosis of such a trend. "Reminiscence spaces" are rooms decorated in the style of the 1950s: newspapers of the time arranged on a bar of the time, old frames, tables and chairs of the time, associated music (Charles Trenet, Edith Piaf), and so on. These initiatives are based on the assumption that older people will be better able to feel at ease in this material environment and that those with dementia will be appeased in this setting, as even when their short-term memory wavers, their long-term memory persists. But most of these activities are based on a set of assumptions regarding the preferences of the elderly. For example, a nursing home staff member tells me that during her "news" activity, she selects only local news, since "at their age" residents are no longer interested in national news and even less in international events. I realize later that she also sought to avoid conflicts that may emerge from news items that may be considered too "political." The gender of the patients can also be the subject of such assumptions. It is agreed among professionals that beauty and body care significantly improve the mental state of female patients, as can be seen in the following extract from an interview with Émilie, a nursing home manager in Quebec:

> Here residents do not really let their face get touched, so it's mostly nail polish, but elsewhere, yeah, the staff even braid their hair. There are some ladies, I tell myself, "She's too demented, it'll never work." But it looks like it's still there, the mechanism comes back, even the most agitated ones calm down, as if at that moment it reminds them... like, "Ah, yes, at that time when I went to the hairdresser".... They feel well, as if this remains, no matter the degree of the illness. It remains. "Ah, I like to try a new polish." Even those who stop walking, each time at the beginning we say, "No, with her, it'll never work," but we try and there, surprise, the lady sits, stretches out her arms, relaxes.... That reminds them of before.

Third, and more specifically, people may refer to the patients' former occupations or leisure and to their nations or regions of origin and their associated "culture." For example, interlocutors tend to assume, as most sociologists do, that the profession someone exercised is key to understanding this person and to interacting with them. This assumption provides topics of conversation and tricks to personalize discussions. Unlike some research, such as that conducted by Dobbs et al.,[4] I did not observe direct discrimination due to residents' social position but rather some generalizations about this or that social milieu. Undertaking such reconstitution in this way requires some generalized representation of the social world in which residents appear to have evolved. Social roles, especially those established and performed in the patient's family, are often underscored: "It is your daughter who comes to see you," "you are happy when your sister visits you, right?" and "she always enjoyed spending time with her family," and so on.

Thus, recalling Mrs. Sinclair, who ran a photography store as a younger woman, we can recognize that both the professionals and her daughter established and maintained an interaction with her by behaving in a manner premised on her belonging to three groups: "normal," through the insistence upon certain greetings and modes of politeness and the assumption that she would like to participate in an activity; women, through the assumption that she wanted to be beautiful; and photographers, who would supposedly appreciate being the subject of a photographic medium.

Reconstitution activities take place at the first signs of the disease and then gradually intensify. Those acquainted with the patient then begin to draw on their knowledge of the patient's past to fill the widening gaps of the present. In the context of nursing homes, this reconstitution becomes institutionalized. Professionals sometimes glean information from relatives and medical records about the past of residents, information that they introduce into interactions in order to refine their reconstitution. In the institutions observed in France and Quebec, specific mechanisms existed to record such information. These were the "Aloïs factsheets" and the "life history binders." But relatively few professionals consulted these documents or knew that they existed. Professionals learn more from varied deductions arising from informal conversations with family members or in corridors or from exchanges with colleagues or executives. These reconstructions can be divided into three categories corresponding to three uses, and it is to these categories that we now turn.

Reconstituting to Understand

[A manager of a Canadian nursing home]
We had an issue with a resident, Mrs. Lien. She was stealing everything around her: towels, tissue packs, food, anything she could take but especially, above all, shoes. All sorts of shoes. Even men's shoes. We had difficulties with that because residents and families were complaining of losing items. Some residents were barefoot! And every time we clean rooms, we find so many things hidden in her bathroom, under her mattress, I don't know ... even under the carpet. But once we did this interdisciplinary meeting with her family. They told us her story. She is like Cambodian or Vietnamese, and she was a young mother when there was a war, something with Khmers. ... Anyway, she had to run away from home. That woman, she was something! She crossed like a thousand kilometers with nothing, not even shoes! No money! No food! And with her two kids! That's

> unbelievable, hey? Now, she looks like . . . so weak. . . . And during
> this meeting, her children emphasized shoes. . . . So when we [the
> staff members] discovered that, that made much more sense. She
> probably had to steal a lot of things to survive. Suddenly, something
> inside of me just clicked: her habit, stealing shoes, it makes much
> more sense now.

Facing behaviors that they do not understand among residents, professionals may retrieve information about the patient's past to make sense of the patient's present behaviors. The case of Mrs. Lien is somewhat striking since we move from a conduct perceived as odd (stealing items and especially shoes) to a conduct perceived as meaningful. I observed the same form of interpretative process toward other patients. Mrs. Simard, for example, would knock at each door of her unit every day, as if she were doing some sort of "rounds." She sometimes even entered the rooms of other residents, which regularly provoked conflict with them. Staff members linked this behavior to her former job. She had been a postwoman. As a nursing assistant told me, "She maybe thinks she is delivering letters." Among some staff members, these hypothetical links between the past and the present become a reasoning pattern, a habit of mind. Thus, when a resident repeatedly entered a manager's office where I was sitting and put the wire of my cell phone charger in his mouth, some reflections emerged among those professionals present. The reflections took the form of a joke but, crucially, in doing so, denoted an attempt to link past and present to demystify the behavior. Was he a former electrician? Did he like to do crafts?

Referring to residents' pasts to understand their behaviors constitutes an efficient interpretive technique, all the more so since the effectiveness of professional activities always remains unclear. This is because the emotional and cognitive states of the patients prevent staff members from knowing clearly whether, and to what extent, their activities have an effect. An example of this occurred when a multisensory space (or "Snoezelen space") was installed in a French nursing home. A multisensory space is a room fitted with a set of supposedly relaxing elements: a massage chair, lighting effects, an essential oil diffuser, relaxing music, "antistress" objects, and so forth. The aim is to help people suffering from dementia to relax. When this space was established, professionals received theoretical training. However, they were not fully confident about the potential of this space and so carried out some "experiments" with a few residents. One staff member chose to bring Mrs. Breton in. Mrs. Breton posed numerous difficulties for the staff since she walked continuously and consequently required constant attention. Successfully calming her would greatly alleviate the staff members' workload and the risk of accident. Because she was the wife of a former head of surgery in the nearby hospital, the staff members associated her with all things "upper class." In the multisensory space, where playing music is recommended, the nursing aide selected a CD that she considered to be within proximity to the musical tastes associated with the "upper class"—namely, classical music. She thus played an album of Ludovico Einaudi. During the session, the resident did indeed calm down, stopped walking and talking, sat on the massage chair, and finally seemed to rest. Commenting on this (exceptional) reaction afterward, the employees explained such success by pointing out Mrs. Breton's familiarity with classical music but also more broadly with this balneotherapy-like configuration. Given her former social milieu, one of them said, "She has probably used to being in these kinds of places."

In addition to activities, using information about residents' pasts may provide professionals with some insights into understanding special relationships. By special relationships, I mean these frequent moments where a resident suddenly displays a special attachment to someone. Thus, on numerous occasions, as I was passing through the communal rooms or corridors of facilities under observation, some residents looked at me with emotion, as if they knew me, as if I was one of their old acquaintances, even coming to talk to me, to take my hand or my arm, and to stare at me closely. They often communicated this disturbing feeling of being strongly connected to me, despite being unable to exchange even a few coherent words. In France as well as in Quebec, professionals who observed such interactions reacted in exactly the same way. The professionals supposed that I reminded the patient of someone whom he or she must have known well, such as their husband or their son. Given that I am pretty tall, the staff sought someone among the resident's (former) acquaintances who was as tall as me or who looked like me more generally. When this kind of situation occurred with female patients, the staff wondered if the patient's son or husband resembled me. If not, staff would joke, saying that perhaps the resident had had an affair with a tall man.

But these associations may be directly suggested by what residents say or do. Mrs. Revel, who often came to see me, addressed me as if I was either her son ("did you do your homework?") or her husband ("darling, are we going out tonight?"). This "role-playing" is sometimes related to the patient's former job:

> [Field notes, Montreal] I am sitting on a chair in front of a table, in an office in a unit specializing in Alzheimer's care. I have left the door open, waiting for a nursing aide whom I am going to interview. A resident passing by in the corridor sees me and enters the room. She greets me and asks me if I am "his brother." I answer that I am not. "I was expecting his mother, but anyway." Looking at my Dictaphone and the consent form on the desk and at the notebook in my hand (I was preparing for the interview with the nursing aide), she sits in front of me. "Well, how do I put this . . . I asked to meet you because this is a place where people work, as you see. But these people have private lives too! If you are late, you can call me, that's okay. But I can't wait after seven p.m. I have kids to care for too. I have to go to collect them, you got it? So, after seven p.m., I really have to leave, understood? [I acquiesce. Silent moment.] So, welcome here! You will study, learn a lot of things about . . . the world. Have you seen all the rooms yet? You will see, going to school is . . . [Looking again to my Dictaphone] Oh, maybe you already know some things. I have to go, bye."

According to the nursing aide who finally arrived, this woman used to "work in a school." In the reported interaction, the female patient seemed to move from the role of a teacher asking a pupil's relative not to be late collecting a child from school to one of a teacher welcoming a new pupil. However, I did not understand the last sentence. Perhaps the recorder enabled her to imagine that I was a teacher myself? Or perhaps maybe this sentence did not mean anything coherent. . . .

Making sense of some interactions with the help of information regarding residents' pasts is a common technique used in order to understand behaviors that remain cryptic. In the end, no matter how "true" these interpretations are, they still provide a means—if not the only available means—whereby people around the patients cope with the apparent incoherence of some behaviors and thereby "individualize" care through assuming that some of the socialization of the residents persists.

Reconstituting to Act

Sometimes, staff members use what they know or assume of residents' pasts to frame their interventions toward them. We have seen an example of this with the aforementioned case of Mrs. Breton and classical music. Below lies the answer of a specialized educator when I asked him to what extent he found it important to know about the former jobs of residents.

> Yes. Sure. You won't take the same approach with the former director of a company of five hundred employees . . . a man who had, all his life, five hundred people under his orders. Well, in this case . . . when you intervene, you try to enhance his skills, you ask him his opinion before doing something. . . . It helps us a lot to understand the personality of people. I remember there was a former trucker, a truck driver. So, with him, when I had to meet him it was . . . [He straightens up, slightly askew, and speaks louder, strengthening his Quebec accent, which evokes the "working class" way of talking] Now, Roger, come off it! You crossed the line and I'm pissed. [With his usual voice] You see, I talk to him like this [Back to the "working class" way of talking] What d'you want? To get smashed up? You'd better cut the crap now! [With his usual voice] I would never talk like that to Mrs. Tremblay, [speaking gently] who is a former schoolteacher, very coquettish and nice. . . . [With his usual voice, laughing] She wouldn't have understood! So, knowing the former job is a good tool in finding the right level with them. There is another resident, she is the mother of eleven children, she stayed at home her whole life to raise them. Can you imagine, eleven children!? I can't. Her, when she says no, it means no, and she is not impressed by us. If she says no you'd better go away and come back later. She is used to making decisions, and she would never let herself be pushed around.

While most staff members say that they take into account what they know about the residents' pasts in their daily encounters with them, they do not systematize them as much as this specialized educator did. To them, it is mainly one of the most efficient "tricks" for creating diversions. When they have to bathe, feed, or dress residents, especially those who are reluctant, staff members talk with them to "refresh their ideas." This is what a manager explained to me: "When you're like . . . stuck here, when you can almost do nothing by yourself and strangers feed you and wash you every day, well it can be humiliating, you know what I mean . . . so it's better when they [staff members] help them feel comfortable, when they make them think of nice things, other things."

In this frame, staff members relate that learning things about a resident's past provides them with easy topics of conversation. For instance, a nursing home assistant said that "there is a resident who liked to fish, so I talk about fish when I give him a bath. Another resident is very interested in her children, so I talk about that with her . . . these kinds of things." These "kinds of things" have proved to be very convenient in fostering the acceptance of care with "difficult" residents. A nursing aide recounted that with Mr. Marcos, a former carpenter, talking about wood was the only way of generating a reaction and of encouraging him to take a bath: "As I come from a region where there are many, many, many woods, I know things, and with him I can talk about wood. [Mimicking] 'Hey, Mr. Marcos, imagine the smell and the feel of oak wood. . . .' [Back to his usual voice] And sometimes, sometimes, I see something in his eyes, I am sure it's doing something to him. . . . I have no proof, but I feel it."

Another example, perhaps surprising, has been observed in France as well as in Canada. Some residents are former train drivers, the knowledge of which staff members utilize in interacting and behaving with them. Staff members talk to them about trains, about travelling with them on trains, and even imitate the noise of a train, all of which helps to render these residents more accommodating.

Creating diversions, though, is above all a manner of dealing with potentially embarrassing situations. Very frequently, some residents think that a relative will soon come to take them back home. In these cases, professionals tell the patients to sit down and to wait for their relatives, pretending that they will come in one hour or two, as residents forget fairly quickly what they were waiting for and move on. Here, references to the patients' pasts are useful in diverting their interest; after a few moments, patients think they were just chatting with a staff member.

Another recurrent occasion where creating a diversion may be useful occurs when residents ask a professional for something (for instance a glass of water) and then forget they have done so. They may ask for the same thing ten times. This occasionally happened to me with Mrs. Breton, the woman who oscillated between thinking that I was her husband and her son. She appreciated "going for a walk" with me, which, in the context of the nursing home, meant strolling around the table in the ward. But at the end of each round, she forgot we had just done a lap of the table and so would ask me to join her on a stroll once more. Once, after our fifteenth round, I was trying to explain to her that I had other things to do—I actually had nothing in particular to do except observe, but this situation made me feel very uncomfortable—when a staff member came up to me. "Look at how I do it," she said. And she began a discussion with Mrs. Breton about her son. Mrs. Breton answered that her son was very bright at school. The staff member suggested she sit down, and she agreed without hesitation.

With residents who are very reluctant to receive care or are bedridden, staff members test different procedures until one of the procedures works. The following interaction shows this process at work. A nurse and a psychologist try to convince a resident, lying on her bed, to try a new wheelchair. They want to get some cooperation from her in order to avoid using more physical means.

Nurse [enthusiastic tune, while the psychologist gently puts her arm around Mrs. Manet's back to straighten her up]: Come on, Mrs. Manet, we need you to make an effort. We'll sit on a new chair! It's going to be much more comfortable!

[Mrs. Manet shouts. She seems sad. The psychologist withdraws her arm.]

Psychologist [she stands right in front of Mrs. Manet, smiling, speaking very softly]: Would you like to take my hand? Will you take my hand?

[Mrs. Manet shouts again. The nurse caresses her arm to try to calm her.]

Nurse: So, are we going?

[The psychologist tries to take Mrs. Manet's hand. The resident screams even louder and slaps the hand of the psychologist. Both professionals take a step backward.]

Psychologist [to the nurse]: I'll try something. [She takes Mrs. Manet's hand while placing her face right in front of Mrs. Manet's eyes, probably to make sure Mrs. Manet sees her well] Mrs. Manet, what does your son do? He's a lawyer, right?

Nurse: I think so. . . .

Psychologist [indicates to the nurse, with a nod, that they can try again to move Mrs. Manet]: Whatever, okay. Think of your son! Do you like when he comes to see you?

[They start to raise Mrs. Manet, but she starts screaming a little louder. They agree to try again the next day.]

If evoking the past or an aspect of the residents' lives can be a means of diverting them, it may also be a means of helping them focus. During a gymnastics activity, residents had to take a stick in their right hand and make it rotate like a metronome. Mrs. Simard, the former postwoman, was experiencing difficulties understanding the activity instructions, and a staff member exclaimed, "Come on, Mrs. Simard! It's like driving a postal car! Left! Right! Left! Right!" At the weekly quiz, special attention was given to Mr. Malus, a resident described by the staff as "someone very, very wise"—he had run the pharmacy in the nearest town. When nobody could answer a question, the activity director asked for Mr. Malus's opinion, publicly marking his past status as a person "who knows things," although he often took this opportunity to make dubious jokes.

When professionals implement collective strategies—sometimes called "action plans"—in order to help residents feel less "anxious" or be less agitated, it happens that they take the gender or the former occupation into account. The psychologist of the French facility told me that one of her greatest successes concerned Mrs. Brunel, a very old woman who was in an advanced stage of dementia but, according to the psychologist, abnormally anxious. Talking with Mrs. Brunel's family, she realized that Mrs. Brunel had been very "coquettish" when she was younger. Therefore, the psychologist suggested staff members regularly perform beauty treatments on her (applying makeup, giving her a manicure, or paying more attention to her clothes and jewelry). Apparently it worked very well; the resident seemed to be calmer and quieter. The specialized educator at a Canadian facility told me about another case where it was quite impossible to bathe a resident. Looking at the resident's life story binder, he remembered that birds fascinated this man. The educator decided to print pictures of birds and put them into frames. He then placed these pictures in the resident's room, tracing a "route" from his bed to the bathroom. In this manner, staff members could make the process of bathing more pleasant for the resident, having more obvious supports for diversions. It apparently worked.

Finally, framing interactions through residents' pasts appears to be necessary when they are migrants, given that as the disease evolves, migrants tend to gradually forget the language of their host country in favor of their mother tongue. Sometimes, migrants forget the language of their country of origin and remember only the dialect of their hometown. Even their family members then experience difficulties in talking with them. Aside from interaction issues, language issues result from historical changes in migration waves in both countries of this study. In France, staff members were drawn from France, Maghreb, and Western Africa; and in Quebec, staff members had origins in the Middle East, Latin America, and the Caribbean. In both cases, this contrasted with the older generation of residents, who in the French context were drawn from Central and Southern Europe and in the Québécois context had their origins in Greece, Italy, and Armenia. This contrast sometimes limits mutual understanding, and some professionals try to adjust themselves to these situations. For example, some professionals attempt to learn foreign words, communicate through hand gestures, or deploy relatively "universal" expressions such as "*manjare*" for "eat"—a translation that works in several languages. Given that in both France and Quebec many staff members learned some Spanish in high school, they often attempt to use Spanish words in speaking with Italian residents, as these two languages share an etymological history and also bear a phonetic resemblance.

In this set of interactions, reconstituting residents' pasts provides the staff members and relatives with a frame for refining their course of action. Staff members may then, for example, turn an initial interaction (such as a bath) into another past-related one (a pleasant stroll among bird pictures or a conversation about trains). These activities thus reinforce the weight of some aspects of the residents' pasts in the present.

Avoiding Reconstitution to Maintain Order

In some rarer situations, references to the past are not as consensual as in the previous examples; staff members generally "unframe" these references to the past in order to manage the institutional routine. I will now review these possibilities.

When they consider that residents could disturb other residents or the institutional order by "reenacting" their pasts, staff members try to stop the patients through diversions. Mr. Tampani, who used to own an Italian restaurant, provides an interesting example. According to a nursing aide, after Mr. Tampani's institutionalization, he recognized the facility's shift changes, the main one of which occurs around 3:00 p.m. Every day, Mr. Tampani would systematically pick up the chairs in the communal rooms of the unit and put them on the tables, as staff in restaurants do at the end of service. Professionals would then go to talk to him, making him think of other things (thereby creating a diversion) so that he would not disturb the whole ward layout. As the disease progresses, patients tend to confuse objects and people. One resident was a former garage owner, and according to a staff member, he spent "three-quarters of his time in his garage," leaning over his bed as if he was examining a car, screwing and unscrewing the mechanical components or spark plugs he imagined he could see. But after a while, he began to think that some residents were motors and tried to move them from their beds, which led professionals to encourage him to stop thinking he was still in his garage. Mrs. Romain had a similar issue. She used to own a tourist lodge with her husband and frequently asked staff members when her husband would be coming to take her back there. Initially, professionals used to simply create a diversion. But she started to associate her dead husband with one another resident in the facility. Worried about the maintenance of her travel lodge and the health of her dogs, she went to this other resident's room while he was sleeping and slapped him to wake him up, asking him to drive her to the lodge.

In such cases, unlike in the previous section, professionals use diversions to take residents away from their memories, as the resurgence of these memories disturbs the institutional order.

Particular elements of the past, in and of themselves, can prove problematic for the maintenance of the institutional order. This is the case of war memories or other associated events, which particularly agitate some residents. "You know what we would say in my family? Well, that there's some deportation in the air! It's a familiar environment," Mrs. Jankevitch said one morning, ironically, regarding institutional life. Obviously, she wanted to shock her companions, and she succeeded in doing so, necessitating an employee intervention: "Come on, Mrs. Jankevitch, do not say this kind of thing." Christophe, the specialized educator, recounted to me a situation that had occurred when he'd gone to the garden of his facility to play ball with some residents. One of the residents suddenly began to shout in Greek, having some kind of panic attack. Nobody understood what was happening. It so happened that a Greek employee of a nearby shop was passing and, in hearing the man shouting, approached the group. The shop employee was able to explain that the resident thought the ball was a grenade. Investigating afterward, the staff member realized that this resident had been a soldier during the Second World War and that he probably experienced flashbacks of the war when they played in the garden. He consequently advised other staff members to "take care" with balls and projectile-like objects.

Some past-related behaviors seem to be even more complicated to manage and require institutional reorganization.

Every morning, Mr. Wong, a former doctor, walks around the ward of the facility. With no doctor's gown or stethoscope, he tries to ensure that each patient has been well diagnosed and has been prescribed the correct medicine. He takes this opportunity to offer medical information and to give advice regarding the day-to-day management of illnesses. Staff members are worried about the consequences of his "rounds": he diagnoses residents with new diseases and makes them doubt their drugs. Nobody succeeds in changing Mr. Wong's mind. When staff members try to do so, he accuses them of being "in denial." They therefore plan to move him to a smaller unit that less resembles a hospital, hoping that this new environment will prevent him from continuing his "medical rounds." Such resurgences are not problematic in themselves for staff members. Mrs. Paquette, a former nurse who, at times, considers herself to be "on duty" has been authorized to attend the staff meetings, as long as she does not disturb anything.

References to past social position take a different connotation when they are used by residents in order to "minimize" the consequences of their impairments. Mr. Jacquot, a sixty-eight-year-old former engineer, caused concern for professionals on account of his propensity for violence. Barely coherent when he talks, he spends his time wandering in the ward. One day he caused some trouble by hitting an employee. Afterward he came to see me in a communal room, trying to explain himself despite his difficulty finding his words.

> I ... I ... I apologize ... all this ... I lose my ... sheep ... oh ... string ... oh ... I'm ill ... up there [indicating his head with his hand] ... when ... I'd like ... ah ... that's life ... the ... the other there ... if you have the time ... my number ... if after ... you do [he stares at his left leg] ... and we can ... grid ... no ... pray ... no ... oh, I apologize ... I was younger ... maths ... I did repair things ... I've done mathematics! Something ... What have I become?

Since these references are justifications and have no consequence on his behavior, professionals may listen sympathetically, but such explications will not influence the professional's course of action in response. Mr. Jacquot was given more medicine and transferred to another ward.

Framing references to the past can also raise vivid negotiations and even conflicts between staff and residents. In both France and

Quebec, I have observed that some female residents enjoy taking care of dolls. According to staff members, the dolls focus their attention and relieves their stress. When walking through common rooms in nursing homes, it is not unusual to see old women taking care of dolls the whole day. While staff members introduce the dolls because they can calm the residents down, introducing the dolls can also create problems later on. Families, and husbands in particular, are generally shocked to see their relative with a doll. It somehow infantilizes the patient and, to husbands, perhaps even "unfeminizes" their wives, whose attitudes and bodies are already affected by their disease. For instance, a nursing assistant told me of the case of a resident whose husband was upset, since the resident increasingly preferred to give her attention to her doll rather than communicate with him. He told the manager that it was unacceptable to encourage his wife's "regressing," and at each visit he threw the doll in the garbage, but staff members took it back after he left. For the staff members, the toy was too important because it prevented the resident from feeling "anxiety." The staff members attempted to make the husband accept this practice, unframing for him references to childhood associated with caring for dolls and explaining that it was a "therapeutic," even a "medical" issue. In other cases, residents caring for dolls seem to relive their mothering responsibilities. Some such residents therefore refuse to eat and drink unless their "child" eats and drinks first, sometimes spilling food and drink on their doll, making a mess on themselves, the doll, and the floor. When it comes to this kind of issue, staff members hesitate before taking dolls back. However, in a Canadian ward they have found a practical trick: they tell the resident that the baby has to sleep because he is too tired to eat and put the doll on the bed during mealtimes.

Conclusion

Since the 1980s, social scientists have mainly conceptualized dementia as a *loss of self*. This conceptualization implies that, following the decline of cognitive abilities, the *self* of ill persons tends to decline little by little. Much research has asked to what extent elderly people who suffer from dementia, or from any kind of cognitive disability, preserve their "identity" or their *self*[5]—for example, by pursuing certain activities that are meaningful for them. In this context, how can one provide assistance to the elderly, affected person experiencing this apparent loss of self? The vision that emerges from such a description of the effects of dementia—namely, the possession and subsequent loss of a sense of self—is limited by its reliance upon a binary construction. Whereas the proponents of an approach in terms of "loss" or "preservation" of "self" generally claim that they oppose an overly mechanical, determinist, and functionalist view of aging, this conceptualization runs the risk of reproducing the same conceptual blockages. They risk encountering four blockages:

First, this conception situates the person on a single axis, on which the self is *more or less* lost or preserved—an axis on which each person around the patients assists them *more or less* in this task of preservation. My observations suggest, on the contrary, that cognitive disorders produce variable and unequal modifications in the conception persons have of themselves and of their actions. Let us take memory. Patients do not uniformly forget, or "lose," each dimension of their pasts and their "identities." Some forget what their former jobs were while they remember which hobbies they used to have; some do not recognize their spouses anymore while they still react to seeing their children. Furthermore, some seem to "relive" parts of their pasts[6]—for instance, occasionally believing that they are on holiday with their parents when they are institutionalized or that their children are going to take them back home. In these cases, health professionals and family caregivers may then encourage some degree of resurgence or may pay no attention to some resurgences while discouraging others. There is no question of "getting lost" in general but one of losing or preserving each element of the past at varying levels, depending on different logics, from preserving the interaction order to trying to make sense of incoherent behaviors.

Second, a common, underlying assumption regarding dementia and aging—as implied by analyses in terms of loss of self—is that the elderly would *systematically* want to preserve, by any means, *what they were before.* This hypothesis seems comprehensible in view of the incapacities sometimes caused by advancing age and cognitive disorders. But what do we really know? Historians of the Second World War have shown that some veterans, who never spoke of what they had experienced during the war, begin to recall their memories as dementia symptoms progress.[7] This suggests that bringing people back to their pasts is not always a matter of preserving their supposed "identity" but is instead to integrate a new facet of their pasts into their daily lives. Furthermore, some may prefer not remember some elements of their "identities" that are too embarrassing or shameful. I once met a resident in the lobby of a facility who boasted of smoking marijuana when he was young and wished to continue, but nobody helped him on account of the deviance associated with recreational marijuana consumption. Life is not a linear and positive set that everyone seeks to "preserve" as they grow older. If we hope that aging is no longer to be a painful decline in which individuals cling to their past pride but a potentially rich and enriching stage of life, then the possibility of evolutions and ruptures, at any age, should first be collectively acknowledged.

Third, the possibility to "preserve" one's "identity" depends on the interactions and physical frameworks that people have access to. By encouraging patients to remember certain things and not others, to relive certain moments and not others, the people around them play a significant role through reconstitution activities. But while the literature on the subject focuses on the posture of the caregivers, on their *efforts* to promote the preservation of "identities," we have seen that other parameters come into play. The first parameter relates to the way in which the resurgences of the past fit into the daily organization of the home or institution and if they facilitate or disrupt the interaction order. Hence, the material context and its management influence reminiscences, especially when this context evokes the patient's previous occupation. This was illustrated with the example of residents who worked in the medical sector and thus found themselves in a relatively familiar environment when they were institutionalized. It should be noted, as a second parameter, that the observations reported in this chapter more abundantly displayed residents who have had "emblematic" occupations, in terms of the objects associated with the profession: train drivers, postmen, and carpenters seem to be more inspiring than those who were doing "something in an office" or "administrative jobs" (an important part of the population that is not represented in the previous observations). Residents who have run their own businesses are also overrepresented, possibly due to the emotional "identity" investment implied by the responsibility of a company. Let us also take into consideration a third parameter—namely, the representation that caregivers have of the social world and the characteristics they associate with each group represented. Let us think of Mrs. Breton and her supposed familiarity with balneotherapy; let us also consider the case of Mrs. Simard and her supposed ability to drive a post office car; and, indeed, let us not forget Roger the trucker and his supposed inclination to communicate abruptly.

Finally, we observed the following social configuration: caregivers, whether professionals or family members (though the former have consumed this chapter's attention), seek to show deference to people who can no longer communicate in the usual ways. To do this, caregivers produce reconstruction activities that lead the interaction to rely upon a certain representation of aging and of the social space.[8] In so doing, depending on the cognitive troubles of the patient, the material context, and the possibilities of interpretation, caregivers favor the preservation of certain elements of the past and not others.

As the social experience of dementia implies becoming gradually the "object" of reconstitution activities, the associated representations (that people use to proceed to reconstitution) increasingly permeate everyday interactions, and by extension, I assume, they permeate the patients' sense of self.

CONCLUSION

W E ARE ALL CAUGHT IN A SET OF interactions that require
constant control of our gestures, our words, our affects, and
the ordinary skills that organize social life—in our relationships
with the people we meet; in demonstrating our ability to recognize
people; to know where we are, when, and with whom; to find our
way around various places; to manage our schedules and appointments. In all of these mundane activities, we find ourselves in the
grips of this controlling modality, this imperative to regulate and
monitor our conduct at all times.

In this ongoing exercise that is never completely successful, we
all oscillate between getting lost and finding ourselves, between
forgetting and remembering. When such oscillation persists, the
interactions that we experience change lastingly. People presenting
troubles associated with a form of dementia have in common this
altered experience of ordinary relations, whose observation allows
"unveiling" some tacitly accepted rules. In other words, the materials of their experience are made of common interactions, progressively altered. Patients must then face with increasing intensity a
different way of being the subject of repairing exchanges, discreditation, deference, and reconstitution.

While Alzheimer's disease, or any other form of dementia, is
experienced as a personal, intimate, cognitive experience, this experience is shaped socially, even collectively. Beyond the peculiar
relations between patients and the people around them, a common
structure "operates." This does not mean that we are doomed to
see this structure repeating itself again and again. For example,
even as this book aims at documenting the "average" experience
of Alzheimer's disease, some social movements are currently questioning interaction patterns surrounding the patients, trying to
construct alternative experiences of the disease. Thus, quite the

contrary, the perspective proposed in this book questions the historical possibilities of change: by showing what is contingent in existing interactions, it becomes possible to ask how the experience of dementia *is contingent* and thus how it could be different.[1] This is why I will conclude with some "historical" remarks.

The Emergence of a Social Role

First, let us observe the growing autonomization of what I call the social role of the elderly living with dementia. The notion of social role refers to the norms and expectations that surround a person when they hold a certain status or engage in a certain activity—for example, the roles of father or mother, spouse, and coworker.[2] We learn these roles gradually, sometimes without thinking, sometimes preparing ourselves, in much the same way that actors adopt characters before entering the scene.

Until recently, elderly people with memory loss or other disorders associated with dementia experienced a gradual deterioration in their previous social roles. They were parents, workers, and aging spouses on the decline, who were therefore asked "a little less."[3] Social expectations were relaxed and diminished. This can be observed in historical and literary works depicting aging before the second half of the twentieth century. The figures of the old man "who loses his mind," of the grandmother who has become "a little crazy," are not new. Discussed by Galen in first-century Greece, staged by Shakespeare more than 1,500 years later in England, formalized by Esquirol in nineteenth-century France, the association between aging and decreasing cognitive abilities unfolds some papyrus at least since antiquity.[4]

My study, however, shows that people considered to be experiencing the effects of dementia do not exactly experience a *loosening* of expectations associated with their previous social roles, except perhaps at the very beginning of their illness trajectory. Rather, they tend to be given a different *total* social role in the sense that they can no longer act (as spouses, relatives, friends, etc.) without those around them wondering to what extent their behavior arises from the disease or to what extent they may represent a domestic danger.

In the field of dementia, the expression of "ambiguous loss" or "social death,"[5] which is even more striking in French (*deuil blanc*, literally "white mourning"), expresses that, at an advanced stage of the disease, people around the patient go through a mourning process while their relative is still alive. She or he is *no longer the same person*, as we hear frequently among caregivers. In other words, the social role of the elderly living with dementia tends to outweigh the other available social roles in quite a definitive fashion.[6]

Logically, the role of "caregiver" follows the same process. Previously, this role was constituted by the declination of one's existing social role, from a spouse, daughter or son, or brother or sister to one who cares for their loved one. Now, this role too becomes autonomous, total in the sense that it tends to permeate all the other roles. The training given for "becoming a caregiver" in some community associations, and the published textbooks on this topic, are two examples among others: it is no longer only a question of principally being a member of the family. People feel the necessity to acquire certain skills, to become adept at ways of doing, and at an organization of life that appears radically different from that of before.

The emergence of a relatively new and autonomous social role, that of the elder living with dementia and the associated caregiver role, reduces the complexity of the previous social existences. Indeed, social roles offer models of behavior that translate an infinite number of questions into a relatively limited set of images, social expectations, and rituals. *We move from a case-by-case organization to a collective scenario.*

Most social roles undergo a similar movement. Let us consider, for example, those of mother or father. Many have long disputed the specificity of these designations: psychologists, educators, teachers, members of associations, and political activists try to define what a parent is, what distinguishes a "good parent" from a "bad parent," a "parent" from a "friend," and a "father" from a "mother." In attempting to do so, each interested party documents, writes, and explains the expected behaviors through educational manuals, laws setting out legal responsibilities, or institutional devices aimed at separating parents who do not meet these expectations from their children.[7] Social roles, initially vague sets of expectations vaguely expressed in some interactions, are made explicit and formal, and sometimes transgressing these expectations puts the transgressors at risk of institutionalized sanctions.

We can find the ferments of the same process with the roles of the elderly suffering from dementia and their caregivers: expectations toward what the disease is and how it should be faced are made more and more explicit, debated, formalized, and *distinguished from the common thread of life.*

But the social role of the elderly person living with dementia has a notable peculiarity: it develops through an insoluble tension. On the one hand, we are seeing the development of specific mechanisms intended to accompany this specific role, such as specialized professional services, specialized institutions, specialized research, and so on. On the other hand, these devices present an ideal according to which the patients remain people like all others. From health professionals to the media, from family associations to public policy makers, all claim that patients are to be treated as "human beings" first and foremost. To do this, and this is where the tension lies, they advocate measures and devices that are increasingly adapted— that is to say, specific, differentiated, and therefore differentiating:[8] this social role has the specificity of being often presented as nonspecific.

Historical Horizons

For this social role to emerge, certain historical conditions have to converge. I will sketch these as an opening, because these go beyond the scope of my research. For example, the social roles of elderly persons living with dementia and the associated caregivers would not take the same form, or even exist, if neoliberal economic policies in the West had not placed an increasing set of pressures on professionals working in the areas of health and aging. These pressures have led professionals to experience a degree of inability with regard to meeting the expectations of patients and families and the values that such parties uphold. As the growing private health sector and the overall bureaucratization of professional activities illustrates, compensating this inability with the standardization of behaviors is a key structuring process in the field of dementia. The social roles in question would not follow the same logic if the public order in our societies did not rely on a principle of self-control and autonomy, or, if there were no such cultural imperatives posing the necessity to justify and express, with the languages of compassion or security, the constraints placed on people who are cognitively different. These roles would certainly not have the same substance without the monopoly exercised by medical representations in the conception of diseases. These roles would not trigger the same collective work without this common conception of the individual as a long-term, coherent, continuous entity whose "personality" must be maintained at all costs, including when cognitive impairment occurs.

This is probably a historical turning point in terms of aging and health. Suffering from a form of dementia is becoming less and less an "on the job" adjustment process but is becoming increasingly experienced a series of preestablished steps and behavioral models, in the sense of being established prior to the emergence of any individual disorders.[9] The proposed sociological perspective thus enables us to examine the historical "levers" by which the social roles discussed are transformed, especially with regard to *representations*.

In the world of aging and dementia and the related public health policies, there is widespread belief in the importance of producing positive representations of older people, especially those with cognitive impairment. Primarily, we can note with Sarah Lamb[10] that these cultural representations—such as the dominant model of "successful aging"—are in themselves reproducing some values, such as the promotion of productivity, which may not be the most inclusive meanings to build a generalized positive model of aging.

Such representations would establish "good" patterns to be followed. It must be remembered, however, that what is at stake in representations lies not only in their *content*—what is represented—but in the relationship between this content and its *mode of production*: who represents who, and in what context? To take a controversial example, the famous Aunt Jemima's pancake syrup presents a picture on the bottle of a nice African American woman with a friendly smile. However, the continued use of this depiction in the postslavery context made advertising dubious. In other words, what is at issue here is the mode of production of the representation more than its content. The same reasoning applies here with the figure of the smiling elderly that can be found in many advertising and public health media produced in the last decades.

It is enough to raise this point to realize that the producers of representations characterizing the social role of the person suffering from dementia are never the concerned people themselves but actors who have an interest in providing help. Indeed, they are often professionals who not only seek to provide help but in fact have a financial interest in doing so. On the brochures and websites of nursing homes, for example, people diagnosed are often represented positively only through the benevolent help configuration that allows them to be happy, which in fact leads to them being seen principally through the eyes of the actors on whom they depend. Renée Beard interestingly points out the same type of contradiction in the US Alzheimer's disease movement, where the patients are difficultly integrated in this movement as spokespersons:[11] they are more *represented* than they *represent themselves*.

This pattern of *representation by others* prevails today and stems, of course, from a relationship of domination.[12] To suffer from dementia, or at least to be recognized as suffering from it, amounts to entering into multiple relationships in which other people are provided the occasion to exercise a certain form of domination— that is, to represent the sufferer of dementia but also to decide on behalf of the sufferer. Diagnosed persons are gradually sidelined, deprived of the mastery of their material and symbolic conditions of life. If I have given so much room to criticizing the values expressed in the world of health, it is because these values, albeit embodying a certain benevolence, nonetheless attenuate our perception of the power dynamics at work. By veiling these relations of domination with words and images, the emphasis put on values also prevents a real political debate to emerge about the material and symbolic conditions of aging and about life with age-related cognitive disorders. In other words, the veiling of these relations of domination diminishes our collective capacity to produce a space of possible behaviors, of possible options, necessary to act on these configurations of domination.

In essence, the crucial issue concerns the lifestyles of the persons diagnosed with dementia and people around them. As long as we do not openly assume the part of control and discreditation that accompanies any form of care and help, we will not be "culturally equipped" to think through the ethical questions that accompany through dementia trajectories, hesitations, and tensions among families and professionals. These questions permeate the complexity of situations and ultimately the lifestyles that are reasonably realizable for patients. In this area, any form of "autonomy" presupposes the possibility of risk; any "benevolence" presupposes stigmatization; any "positive representation" presupposes the *euphemization of a relationship of domination*. This rise in complexity summarizes the political and ethical point of a systematic work of description regarding the interactions surrounding the people diagnosed with dementia. And showing these complexities is a condition for any attempt to widen the panel of possible futures.

NOTES

Introduction

1. Norbert Elias, *The Civilizing Process, Vol. II. State Formation and Civilization* (Oxford: Blackwell, 1982) 233–34.

2. The way in which dementia is represented and shaped as a medical reality has been further developed in many publications. See Margaret Lock, *The Alzheimer Conundrum: Entanglements of Dementia and Aging* (Princeton, NJ: Princeton University Press, 2013); Annette Leibing and Lawrence Cohen, eds., *Thinking about Dementia: Culture, Loss, and the Anthropology of Senility. Studies in Medical Anthropology* (New Brunswick, NJ: Rutgers University Press, 2006). The critical perspective to biomedicalization (which I follow to some extent) has been introduced since the 1980s, when dementia became a "public health problem"—for instance, with Karen A. Lyman, "Bringing the Social Back in: A Critique of the Biomedicalization of Dementia," *The Gerontologist* 29(5) (1989): 597–605.

3. This ethnographic methodological approach relies on both Matthew Desmond, "Relational Ethnography," *Theory and Society* 43(5) (2014): 547–79; and George Marcus, "Ethnography In/of the World System: The Emergence of Multi-Sited Ethnography," *Annual Review of Anthropology* (1995): 95–117.

4. The results of this research have been published in French: Baptiste Brossard, "Un test rudimentaire mais pratique. Enquête sur le succès du *Mini-Mental State Examination*," *Sciences sociales et santé* 32(4) (2014): 43–70; Solène Billaud and Baptiste Brossard, "L'expérience' du vieillissement," *Genèses* (95) (2014): 71–94.

5. The ethnography of nursing homes is a flourishing area of study, especially since the pioneering work of Jaber F. Gubrium, *Living and Dying at Murray Manor* (Charlottesville: University of Virginia Press, 1975); Timothy Diamond, *Making Gray Gold: Narratives of Nursing Home Care*, 1st ed. (Chicago: University of Chicago Press, 1995); and the more recent interest in emotions in institutional settings.

6. In this book, I will use the term "nursing aide" for the professionals who hold the lowest position in the nursing home hierarchy—which facilitates developments valid in multiple countries.

7. I have explicated my position on the issues of interpretation in the following article: Baptiste Brossard, "Situating Words: What Grounded Theory Brings to Dementia Research, and Vice Versa," *Sociological Focus* (January 2019), https://doi.org/10.1080/00380237.2018.1544518. I argue against the two major positions regarding the interpretation of the patients' discourses: taking these discourses as "pure meanings" or "pure symptoms." I suggest that social scientists rather have to help make sense of what people say and of their "credibility configurations."

8. Tom Kitwood grandly contributed to promote investigation in this area from a psychological angle. Tom Kitwood, "The Experience of Dementia," *Aging & Mental Health* 1(1) (1997): 13–22.

9. I herein refer to two "typical" studies of the experience of dementia in the field of dementia studies: Guy Harman and Linda Clare, "Illness Representations and Lived Experience in Early-Stage Dementia," *Qualitative Health Research* 16(4) (2006): 484–502; and Linda Clare, Julia Rowlands, Errollyn Bruce, Claire Surr, and Murna Downs, "The Experience of Living with Dementia in Residential Care: An Interpretative Phenomenological Analysis," *The Gerontologist* 48(6) (2008): 711–72.

10. On cultural variations, see Bianca Brijnath, *Unforgotten: Love and Culture of Dementia Care in India* (New York: Bergham, 2014); and Lawrence Cohen, *No Aging in India: Alzheimer's, The Bad Family, and Other Modern Things* (Berkeley: University of California Press, 1998).

11. This expression refers to Randall Collins, *Interaction Ritual Chains* (Princeton, NJ: Princeton University Press, 2005).

12. This expression refers to Robert M. Emerson and Sharon L. Messinger, "The Micro-Politics of Trouble," *Social Problems* 25(2) (1977): 121–34. Béliard and Eideliman showed particularly well the relevance of this theory in the case of dementia: Aude Béliard and Jean-Sebastien Eideliman, "Words for Ills: Diagnostic Theories and Health Problems," *French Journal of Sociology* 55(3) (2014): 507–36.

13. This nuance distinguishes my approach from the perspective proposed by Gaynord Macdonald, Jane Mears, and Ailin Naderbagi, according to whom "the experience of dementia is social—these brain changes affect a person's behaviour as the capacity for independent social interaction is impaired" (3). Conceptually, they enunciate a direct link between brain changes and behavior changes that *impacts* interaction, preventing interactions from being "independent," whereas in my model the interaction is the medium through which the social experience realizes itself. Gaynord Macdonald, Jane Mears, and Ailin Naderbagi, "Reframing Dementia: The Social Imperative," in *Dementia as a Social Experience: Valuing Life and Care*, ed. Gaynord Macdonald and Jane Mears (New York & London: Routledge, 2018), 1–19.

14. Erving Goffman, "The Interaction Order: American Sociological Association, 1982 Presidential Address," *American Sociological Review* 48(1) (1983): 1–17.

15. Ian Hacking, *The Social Construction of What?* (Cambridge, MA: Harvard University Press, 2000).

16. These comments are notably phrased by Stefan Timmermans and Steven Haas, "Towards a Sociology of Disease," *Sociology of Health and Illness* 30 (5) (2008): 659–76.

17. Drew Halfmann, "Recognizing Medicalization and Demedicalization: Discourses, Practices, and Identities," *Health* 16(2) (2011): 186–207.

18. This conception fundamentally relies on Cooley's theory of the construction of the self in social life [*Human Nature and the Social Order* (New York: Charles Scribner, 1902)].

1. The Organization of Repairing Exchanges

1. Quite logically, online sources of information tend to play a greater role in this quest, and it is likely that in the coming decades we will need more investigations into how the structure of online worlds shape access to information in the area of dementia. For now, see Michael Lawless, Martha Augoustinos, and Amanda Le Couteur, "Dementia on Facebook: Requesting Information and Advice about Dementia Risk-Prevention on Social Media," *Discourse, Context and Media* (February 2018), https://doi.org/10.1016/j.dcm.2018.01.011.

2. Erving Goffman, *Interaction Ritual: Essays on Face-to-Face Behavior* (Garden City, NY: Anchor Books, 1967).

3. Normalization in the sense of Thomas Scheff, "Updating Labelling Theory: Normalizing but Not Enabling," *Nordic Journal of Social Research* 1 (April 26, 2017), https://doi.org/10.7577/njsr.2044.

4. On the notion of dementia as risk, see R. Milne, A. Diaz, S. Badger, E. Bunnik, K. Fauria, and K. Wells, "At, with and beyond Risk: Expectations of Living with the Possibility of Future Dementia," *Sociology of Health and Illness* 40 (2018): 969–87.

5. This focus on observability is inspired by Moreno Pestana's study on anorexia—he deals with the observability of diet among young women—itself referring to the theory of ecological niche proposed by Hacking. Jose-Luis Moreno Pestana, "Un cas de déviance dans les classes populaires: Les seuils d'entrée dans les troubles alimentaires," *Cahiers d'économie et Sociologie Rurales*, 79, 1 (2006): 67–95. Ian Hacking, *Mad Travelers: Reflections on the Reality of Transient Mental Illnesses* (Charlottesville: University of Virginia Press, 1998).

6. Bernard Vaussion and Christian Roudaut, *Au service du palais. 40 ans dans les cuisines de l'Elysée* (Paris: Le poche du moment, 2016).

7. I develop on this point in Baptiste Brossard, "Objectifying Dementia," in *Measuring Mental Disorders*, ed. Philippe Le Moigne (London: ISTE Science Publishing, 2018), 127–54.

8. Laurence Tessier, comparing diagnosis methods in the United States and in France, does not highlight significant differences in diagnostic techniques but rather in the emotions raised by the doctors as being at the core of the symptomatology. Laurence Tessier, "Social Brains: On Two Neuroscientific Conceptions of Human Sociality," *BioSocieties* (May 2018): 1–27, https://doi.org/10.1057/s41292-018-0117-0.

9. The best account of this process surrounding the medical consultation is probably Renée Beard, *Living with Alzheimer's: Managing Memory Loss, Identity, and Illness* (New York: New York University Press, 2016).

10. For instance, R. Nay, M. Bauer, D. Fetherstonhaugh, W. Moyle, L. Tarzia, and L. McAuliffe, "Social Participation and Family Carers of People Living with Dementia in Australia," *Health and Social Care*, 23(5): 550–58.

11. Quinn et al. shows that the biomedical model of disease prevails among the caregivers' representations of dementia. Catherine Quinn, Ian Rees Jones, and

Linda Clare, "Illness Representations in Caregivers of People with Dementia," *Aging & Mental Health* 21(5): 553–61.

12. Lydia Lécher's testimony is quite interesting in this regard. She writes, "In a property where she worked, Lydia was forbidden to walk on the gravel aisles, so that nobody see the trace of her steps, and had to sidestep when Mister arrived, because he did not stand seeing the help." [Lydia Lécher, *Bienvenue chez les riches* (Paris: Michel Lafon, 2016).]

13. Elizabeth Peel and Rosie Harding, "'It's a Huge Maze, the System, It's a Terrible Maze': Dementia Carers' Constructions of Navigating Health and Social Care Services," *Dementia* 13(5) (2013): 642–61.

14. Florence Weber, Séverine Gojard, and Agnès Gramain, *Charges de famille: dépendance et parenté dans la France contemporaine* (Paris: La Découverte, 2003); Aude Béliard, "Des familles bouleversées. Aux prises avec le registre diagnostic Alzheimer" (PhD diss., Université Paris Vincennes Saint-Denis, 2010).

15. By this question, I highlight that the issue of support is not only a matter of what support the patients can get but of what support they allow themselves to seek. This is an underestimated question in the literature, which often assumes too quickly that patients naturally seek support. R.V. Herron and M.W. Rosenberg, "'Not There Yet': Examining Community Support from the Perspective of People with Dementia and Their Partners in Care," *Social Science & Medicine* 173 (2017): 81–87.

16. This is history that, among others, Michel Foucault studied. Michel Foucault, *History of Madness* [New York: Routledge, 2006 (1961)].

17. The most up-to-date account of the relations between dementia and social class is Ian Jones, "Social Class, Dementia and the Fourth Age," *Sociology of Health and Illness* 39 (2017): 303–17.

18. See for instance the literature review proposed by Melanie Luppa, Tobias Luck, Siegfried Weyerer, Hans-Helmut König, and Steffi G. Riedel-Heller, "Gender Differences in Predictors of Nursing Home Placement in the Elderly: A Systematic Review," *International Psychogeriatrics*, 21(6) (2009): 1015–25

19. Solène Billaud, "Partager avant l'héritage, financer l'hébergement en institution: enjeux économiques et mobilisations familiales autour de personnes âgées des classes populaires" (PhD diss., Ecole Normale Supérieure/EHESS, 2010).

20. This has been shown in France by Louis Chauvel, *Le destin des générations. Structure sociale et cohortes en France du XXe siècle aux années 2010* (Paris: Presses Universitaires de France, 2010). But we can find some similar observations in the United States: Karin Kurz and Hans-Peter Blossfeld, eds., *Home Ownership and Social Inequality in Comparative Perspective* (Stanford, CA: Stanford University Press, 2004), chapter 12 in particular.

21. I refer to the convincing conceptual attempts to rethink agency in the case of dementia. Geraldine Boyle, "Recognising the Agency of People with Dementia," *Disability & Society* 29(7) (2014): 1130–44.

22. On family deceits and ruses to discourage elders from engaging in activities perceived as potentially dangerous, see Brandon Berry, Ester Carolina Apesoa-Varano, and Yarin Gomez, "How Family Members Manage Risk Around

Functional Decline: The Autonomy Management Process in Households Facing Dementia," *Social Science & Medicine* 130 (2015): 107–14.

2. Losing Credibility

1. I herein endorse Philip Manning's interpretation of Goffman's work as a study of credibility in interaction. Philip Manning, "Credibility, Agency, and the Interaction Order," *Symbolic Interaction* 23(3) (2000): 283–97.

2. Lara Mahi, "The Sanitization of Criminal Justice? The Use of Illness in Criminal Trials," *French Journal of Sociology* 56(4) (2015): 697–733.

3. For insightful reflections on this particular case, read Laurence Tessier, "Seeing a Brain through an Other: The Informant's Share in the Diagnosis of Dementia," *Culture, Medicine, and Psychiatry* 41(4) (2017): 541–63.

4. Penelope A. Pollitt, "The Problem of Dementia in Australian Aboriginal and Torres Strait Islander Communities: An Overview," *International Journal of Geriatric Psychiatry* 12(2) (1997): 155–63.

5. This specific citation is written in the following synthesis text: Carolina Kobelinsky, "Juger l'homosexualité, attribuer l'asile," December 17, 2015, https://la-viedesidees.fr/Juger-l-homosexualite-attribuer-l-asile.html. For an English account of this study, see Carolina Kobelinsky, "The Moral Judgment of Asylum Seekers in French Reception Centers," *Anthropology News* 49 (2008): 5–11.

6. Sikes and Hall thus talk of "grief-related perceptions." Pat Sikes and Mela-nie Hall, "'Every Time I See Him He's the Worst He's Ever Been and the Best He'll Ever Be': Grief and Sadness in Children and Young People Who Have a Parent with Dementia," *Mortality* 22(4) (2017): 324–38.

7. *Béberre* is a French provincial colloquialism evoking an affable but uncouth man, suggestive of a working-class background.

8. For more detail, see Baptiste Brossard, "Reactions to Discredit in Memory Consultation," *Journal of Contemporary Ethnography* 46(1) (2015): 30–50.

9. Erving Goffman, *The Presentation of Self in Everyday Life* (New York: An-chor, 1959).

10. If we consider diagnosis and low score at cognitive tests as a form of dis-credit. Gavin Turrell, John W. Lynch, George A. Kaplan, Susan A. Everson, Eeva-Liisa Helkala, Jussi Kauhanen, and Jukka T. Salonen, "Socioeconomic Position Across the Lifecourse and Cognitive Function in Late Middle Age," *The Journals of Gerontology: Series B* 57(1) (2002): 43–51; T. Staff, D. Chapko, M. J. Hogan, and L. J. Whalley, "Life Course Socioeconomic Status and the Decline in Information Processing Speed in Late Life," *Social Science & Medicine* 151 (2016): 130–38.

11. Béliard, "Des familles bouleversées."

12. This argument of the benefits of the social proximity with doctors has been greatly addressed in the pioneering study of August B. Hollingshead and Fredrick C. Redlich, *Social Class and Mental Illness: A Community Study* (Hoboken, NJ: John Wiley & Sons, 1958). However, it is still a topic of interest, widely discussed in

sociology of health and the related fields. See for instance Jennifer Malat, "Social Distance and Patients' Rating of Healthcare Providers," *Journal of Health and Social Behavior* 42(4) (2001): 360–72; Chloë Fitzgerald and Samia Hurst, "Implicit Bias in Healthcare Professionals: A Systematic Review," *BMC Medical Ethics* 18 (2017): 19.

13. Pierre Bourdieu, *Distinction: A Social Critique of the Judgement of Taste* (New York: Routledge, 1984).

14. I expand on this question in Brossard, "Situating Words."

15. This methodological problem related to sexuality studies has been addressed in France by Nathalie Bajos and Michel Bozon, *Enquête sur la sexualité en France. Pratiques, genre et santé* (Paris: La Découverte, 2008).

16. Some relatively alternative frames exist, such as the one proposed by disability studies, but they are not popular enough to constitute, *practically*, interpretive alternatives for laypeople.

17. This question arose in the sociology of work, at least since this famous article written by Donald Roy, who shows how factory workers have constructed informal times embedded in prescribed work times decided by the management. Donald Roy, "'Banana Time': Job Satisfaction and Informal Interaction," *Human Organization* 18(4) (1959): 158–68.

18. Some research shows how different explanations are shaped to make sense of "suffering" in the workplace. Marlène Benquet, Pascal Marichalar, and Emmanuel Marin, "Responsabilités en souffrance. Les conflits autour de la souffrance psychique des salariés d'EDF-GDF (1985–2008)," *Sociétés contemporaines* 3(79) (2010): 121–43.

19. Neil J. Henderson and Carson L. Henderson, "Cultural Construction of Disease: A 'Supernormal' Construct of Dementia in an American Indian Tribe," *Journal of Cross-Cultural Gerontology* 17(3) (2002): 197–212.

20. Harriet G. Rosenberg, "Complaint Discourse, Aging and Caregiving among the Ju/'hoansi of Botswana," in *The Cultural Context of Aging: Worldwide Perspectives*, ed. Jay Sokolovsky (Westport, CT: Praeger, 2009), 33–55.

3. The Deference Industry

1. In France, the neologism *bientraitance*—literally "well-treatment"—currently epitomizes this lexicon; ANESM (agence nationale de l'évaluation et de la qualité des établissements et services sociaux et médico-sociaux), *La Bientraitance : Définition et Repères Pour La Mise En Œuvre* (Saint-Denis, France: ANESM, 2008). In Québec, public policies try to make nursing homes a "living environment approach," in French "l'approche milieu de vie"; Daniel Proulx, *Approche milieu de vie en CHSLD : cadre de référence* (Laval: Régie régionale de la santé et des services sociaux de Laval, 1998). In the United States, the expression "culture change movement" or "person-centered care" are privileged; Mary Jane Koren, "Person-Centered Care for Nursing Home Residents: The Culture-Change Movement," *Health Affairs* 29(2) (2010): 312–17.

2. In addition, I suggest that a critique of the notion of humanity is not neces-sarily embedded into some "transhuman" or "posthumanist" framework, as Jen-kins seems to think; Nicholas Jenkins, "No Substitute for Human Touch? Towards a Critically Posthumanist Approach to Dementia Care," *Ageing and Society* 37(7) (2017): 1484–98.

3. Erving Goffman, "The Nature of Deference and Demeanor," *American Anthropologist* 58(3) (1956): 473–502.

4. Alexis de Tocqueville, *Democracy in America* (Chicago: University of Chi-cago Press, 2000), third book, chapter 3.

5. Studies of deference have emerged in many fields of research, precisely be-cause this topic concerns all social groups. Most consist of culturalist analyses, such as Kumagai, who examined the display of affection and deference among Japanese people; Akindele, who studied greetings among the Yoruba of Nigeria; or Lanza-Ka-duce and Greenleaf, who analyzed interactions between police officers and citizens in the United States; Akindele, Femi Akindele, "A Sociolinguistic Analysis of Yoruba Greetings," *African Languages and Cultures* 3(1) (1990): 1–14; Hisa A. Kumagai, "A Dissection of Intimacy: A Study of 'Bipolar Posturing' in Japanese Social Inter-action—Amaeru and Amayakasu, Indulgence and Deference," *Culture, Medicine and Psychiatry* 5(3) (1981): 249–72; Lonn Lanza-Kaduce and Richard G. Greenleaf, "Age and Race Deference Reversals: Extending Turk on Police-Citizen Conflict," *Journal of Research in Crime and Delinquency* 37(2) (2000): 221–36. The notion of deference is also used in several initiatives to advance the "general" sociological theory; William A. Faunce, "On the Meaning of Occupational Status: Implications for Stratification Theory and Research," *Sociological Focus* 23(4) (1990): 267–85; Tim Hallett, "Between Deference and Distinction: Interaction Ritual through Symbolic Power in an Educa-tional Institution," *Social Psychology Quarterly* 70(2) (2007): 148–71. However, almost no author addresses how deferential behaviors are socially and historically produced, except Norbert Elias and a few others, such as Claudine Haroche (2000) and Jeremy Keenan (2003). In this chapter, I try to pursue this historicized perspective of defer-ence and power, focusing on the *production process* of deference rather than on its only characteristics (in comparison, Goffman tends to take a structuralist stance on deference, in the sense that he aims to identify some basic patterns that always occur in all social settings); Elias, *The Civilizing Process*; Claudine Haroche, "Le Comporte-ment de Déférence," *Communications* 69(1) (2000): 5–26; Jeremy Keenan, "Dressing for the Occasion: Changes in the Symbolic Meanings of the Tuareg Veil," *Journal of North African Studies* 8(3–4) (2003): 97–120.

6. Because any institution produces some kind of deference, I will allow myself to compare nursing homes with other facilities or places, in a way inspired by Everett Hughes, whose approach "puts [any social object] in perspective with an as large as possible series of cases, defined by the selection of a particular property. [It] is not used for demonstrative value, but to broaden the reader's (or research-er's) perception by suggesting unusual connections between cases that ordinary perception . . . normally leads to separate." Jean-Michel Chapoulie, "La Concep-tion de La Sociologie Empirique d'Everett Hughes," *Sociétés contemporaines* 27(1) (1997): 97–109.

7. This converges with what Rodriquez observes but formulates in emotional terms: the use of emotions as necessary to provide what is conceived of as "real care" and to foster patients' acceptance of staff members' requests. Jason Rodriquez, "Attributions of Agency and the Construction of Moral Order: Dementia, Death, and Dignity in Nursing-Home Care," *Social Psychology Quarterly* 72(2) (2009): 165–79.

8. Steven H. Lopez, "Emotional Labor and Organized Emotional Care Conceptualizing Nursing Home Care Work," *Work and Occupations* 33(2) (2006): 133–60.

9. Or, this is not a matter of how "utopian ideals" can take the shape of practice; Anthea Innes, *Dementia studies: A Social Science Perspective* (London: Sage, 2009).

10. Clare Stacey, *The Caring Self: The Work Experiences of Home Care Aides* (Ithaca, NY: Cornell University Press, 2011).

11. As François Aubry shows: François Aubry, "La place du groupe de pairs dans l'intégration des nouvelles aides-soignantes dans les EHPAD," *SociologieS*, 2010, https://journals.openedition.org/sociologies/3291.

12. Arlie R. Hochschild, "Emotion Work, Feeling Rules, and Social Structure," *The American Journal of Sociology* 85(3) (1979): 551–75.

13. Sass specifically extends on this range of emotions; James S. Sass, "Emotional Labor as Cultural Performance: The Communication of Caregiving in a Nonprofit Nursing Home," *Western Journal of Communication* 64(3) (2000): 330–58.

14. Furthermore, the arrangements that staff members resort to in order to deal with organizational constraints have also attracted an increasing amount of attention in the nursing home ethnography literature. Deborah Reed-Danahay, "'This Is Your Home Now!': Conceptualizing Location and Dislocation in a Dementia Unit," *Qualitative Research* 1(1) (2001): 47–63; Tove Persson and David Wästerfors, "'Such Trivial Matters': How Staff Account for Restrictions of Residents' Influence in Nursing Homes," *Journal of Aging Studies* 23(1) (2009): 1–11.

15. This distinction is derived from the concepts of primary and secondary frames in Goffman's *frame analysis*. To be more specific, I could have phrased this distinction as between "primary frame institutions" and "secondary frame institutions," a question that goes beyond the scope of the present book. Erving Goffman, *Frame Analysis: An Essay on the Organization of Experience* (Cambridge, MA: Harvard University Press, 1974).

16. This is why I acknowledge the "need to revolutionize residential care," observed by several researchers and professionals, while remaining skeptical about the possibilities to provoke such *actual* change without deep structural reforms. Kristine Theurer, Ben Mortenson, Robyn Stone, Melinda Suto, Virpi Timonen, and Julia Rozanova, "The Need for a Social Revolution in Residential Care," *Journal of Aging Studies* 35 (2015): 201–10.

17. The "authenticity work" that Scott observes among mental health peer support workers can be found in this context as well; Anne Scott, "Authenticity Work: Mutuality and Boundaries in Peer Support," *Society and Mental Health* 1(3) (2011): 173–84.

18. Bernard Ennuyer, *Repenser le maintien à domicile* (Paris: Dunod, 2014).

19. Max Weber, "Bureaucracy," in *From Max Weber: Essays in Sociology*, ed. H. Gerth and C. W. Mills (New York: Oxford University Press, 1947), 196–244.

20. Luc Boltanski and Eve Chiapello, The New Spirit of Capitalism (New York: Verso, 2005).

4. Reconstituting People

1. Anders Næss, Eivind Grip Fjær, and MiaVabø, "The Assisted Presentations of Self in Nursing Home Life," *Social Science & Medicine* 150 (2016): 153–59.

2. Theodore Caplow, "Rule Enforcement without Visible Means: Christmas Gift Giving in Middletown," *American Journal of Sociology*, 89(6) (1984): 1306–23; Nicolas Herpin and Daniel Verger, "Flux et superflu : l'échange des cadeaux en fin d'année," *Economie et statistique* 173(1) (1985): 33–47.

3. Sue Estroff, *Making It Crazy: An Ethnography of Psychiatric Clients in an American Community* (Berkeley: University of California Press, 1981).

4. Debra Dobbs, Kevin Eckert, Bob Rubinstein, Lynn Keimig, Leanne Clark, Ann Christine Frankowski, and Sheryl Zimmerman, "An Ethnographic Study of Stigma and Ageism in Residential Care or Assisted Living," *The Gerontologist* 48(4) (2008): 517–26.

5. The best description of this emerging trend is probably Elizabeth Herskovits, "Struggling over Subjectivity: Debates about the 'Self' and Alzheimer's Disease," *Medical Anthropology Quarterly* 9(2) (1995):146–64. Many subconceptualizations have also emerged in this realm. Let us give a few examples. Vittoria studies how professionals try to preserve the patients' identities through various lines of actions such as "communicative care" and "identity work," alternatively targeting their "storied self," the "new self," and the "imagined self"; Anne K. Vittoria, "Preserving Selves Identity Work and Dementia," *Research on Aging* 20(1) (1998): 91–136. Eustache et al. distinguish "sameness" and "selfhood" in the patients' "sense of identity"; M. L. Eustache et al., "Sense of Identity in Advanced Alzheimer's Dementia: A Cognitive Dissociation between Sameness and Selfhood?" *Consciousness and Cognition* 22(4) (2013):1456–67. Hellström et al. identify three different patterns in diagnosed women living at home: keeping the core of the self through the home, keeping the self through polarizing division of labor, and keeping the self through (re-) negotiations of responsibilities; I. Hellström, H. Eriksson, and J. Sandberg, "Chores and Sense of Self: Gendered Understandings of Voices of Older Married Women with Dementia," *International Journal of Older People Nursing* 10 (2015): 127–35. While differences exist in the various definitions of "identity" or "self" and in the methodology considered to be relevant in studying these notions—interviews with patients, observations, standardized testing, theoretical discussions—all these works tend to move in the same direction: as Caddell and Clare (2010) conclude their review of this huge amount of literature, people suffering from dementia experience both continuity and change in their "sense of identity"; Lisa S. Caddell and Linda Clare, "The

Impact of Dementia on Self and Identity: A Systematic Review," *Clinical Psychology Review* 30(1) (2010): 113–26.

6. Kontos has conducted pioneering work in criticizing the centrality attributed to mind in dementia studies and proposing instead to think of dementia as disturbing the "*embodied* selfhood," the habitus. My observations converge in this sense, since they show how habits acquired all along the life course tend to be preserved through bodily reminiscences. Pia C. Kontos, "Ethnographic Reflections on Selfhood, Embodiment and Alzheimer's Disease," *Ageing & Society* 24(6) (2004): 829–49; Pia Kontos and Wendy Martin, "Embodiment and Dementia: Exploring Critical Narratives of Selfhood, Surveillance, and Dementia Care," *Dementia* 12(3) (2013): 288–302.

7. Andrea Capstick and David Clegg, "Behind the Stiff Upper Lip: War Narratives of Older Men with Dementia," *Journal of War & Culture Studies* 6(3) (2013): 239–54.

8. To endorse Jones's critique of the place attributed to social class in dementia research (inequalities in epidemiology, in diagnosis, and in access to care), here is another mechanism through which social distinctions influence the making of dementia; I. R. Jones, "Social Class, Dementia and the Fourth Age," *Sociology of Health and Illness* 39(2) (2017): 303–17.

Conclusion

1. I agree with McParland et al.'s argument, according to which it is reductive to oppose a "positive" and "negative" experience of dementia, and hope that my perspective—exploring contingency rather than distinguishing between "living well" and "badly" with dementia—contributes to this idea. Patricia McParland, Fiona Kelly, and Anthea Innes, "Dichotomising Dementia: Is There Another Way?" *Sociology of Health and Illness* 39 (2017): 258–69.

2. Here I use the notion of "social role" in its very classical sense, outlined by Linton [*The Cultural Background of Personality* (New York: Appleton-Century-Crofts, 1945)] and refined by Merton ["The Role-Set: Problems in Sociological Theory," *The British Journal of Sociology* 8(2) (1957): 102–20]. In this regard, I associate this notion with the notion of "role-set," but I consider that this distinction is not necessary to be developed in the frame of the present text.

3. In line with Parsons's observations regarding the "sick role"; Talcott Parsons, *The Social System* (Glencoe, IL: The Free Press, 1951).

4. See, for example, François Bollera and Margaret Forbes, "History of Dementia and Dementia in History: An Overview," *Journal of the Neurological Sciences* 158(2) (1998): 125–33; Axel Karenberg and Hans Förstl, "Dementia in the Greco-Roman World," *Journal of the Neurological Sciences* 244(1–2) (2006): 5–9.

5. See in particular Helen Sweeting and Mary Gilhooly, "Dementia and the Phenomenon of Social Death," *Sociology of Health & Illness* 19 (1997): 93–117. This ambiguous representation of patients in the late stages of the disease is also

incarnated in the "inadmissible" desires expressed by some relatives to reach the end of the situation: Mel Hall and Pat Sikes, "'It Would Be Easier If She'd Died': Young People with Parents with Dementia Articulating Inadmissible Stories," *Qualitative Health Research* 27(8) (2017): 1203–14.

6. Maybe the emerging forms of "dementia activism" can be taken as an outcome of this process; R. Bartlett, "The Emergent Modes of Dementia Activism," *Ageing and Society* 34(4) (2014): 623–44.

7. For instance, see the history of child protection in the United States: John Myers, "A Short History of Child Protection in America," *Family Law Quarterly* 42(3) (2008): 449–63.

8. I hope that this conceptualization of dementia as an autonomized social role also offers some leads to go beyond the very simplistic accounts of social participation provided by some research, where social participation is measured by individualized indicators (how people take part in their local community, etc.). See, for instance, Linda Birt, Fiona Poland, Ernese Csipke, and Georgina Charlesworth, "Shifting Dementia Discourses from Deficit to Active Citizenship," *Sociology of Health and Illness* 39 (2017): 199–211.

9. This is the classical definition of a social fact by Émile Durkheim, *The Rules of Sociological Method and Selected Texts on Sociology and Its Method* (New York: Free Press, 1982 [1895]).

10. Sarah Lamb, "Permanent Personhood or Meaningful Decline: Toward a Critical Anthropology of Successful Aging," *Journal of Aging Studies* 29(1) (2014): 41–52.

11. Renée Beard, "Advocating Voice: Organisational, Historical and Social Milieux of the Alzheimer's Disease Movement," *Sociology of Health & Illness* 26 (2004): 797–819.

12. This is a typical mechanism of "symbolic violence" [Pierre Bourdieu, *Language and Symbolic Power* (Harvard University Press: Cambridge, 1991)]. Interestingly, domination has also been conceptualized, about another topic, as a "representation by others" by Edward Said, "Orientalism Reconsidered," *Cultural Critique* 1 (1985): 89–107.

INDEX

Accreditation Canada, xiii, 73, 82
accreditation standards for nursing
    homes, xiii, 73, 81, 82, 96, 99
activities for nursing home residents,
    82, 86–89, 105
alarm systems, 21
Aloïs factsheets, 111
ambiance of nursing homes, 81
ambiguous loss, 129
amyloid plaques, x, 17
anosognosia, 38, 47
assistance, types of, 19–20
assisted self-presentation, 103
autonomy, ix–x, 19–20, 65
avoidance of patients, 21–22

Beard, Renée, 132
beauty and body care, 54–56, 110, 119
Béliard, Aude, 24, 50
belongings of institutionalized
    residents, 31, 32
Billaud, Solène, xi, xiv, 32
bingo games, 86–89, 105
body language and discreditation of
    patients, 40
Boltanski, Luc, 99
Botswana, Ju/'hoansi people, 69
Bourdieu, Pierre, 53
bureaucratization of dementia care, 85,
    99–100, 131

Canadian nursing home accreditation
    standards, xiii, 73, 82
caregiver role, 129–30. See also family
    caregivers
caregiving networks, 19–24
Carpentier, Normand, xiii–xiv, 7

case managers, 22
centralized caregiving networks, 23, 24
Chiapello, Eve, 99
childhood memories, 48, 49–50
Chirac, Jacques, 7–8
clock test, 11
coherence in presentation of self, 39–40
communication difficulties. See
    nonspeaking patients; reconstitution
conflicts within caregiving networks,
    23–24
confusing people with others, 113–14
corrective process, 5
credibility. See loss of credibility
cultural capital and discreditation,
    52–53
culture of origin and relational skills,
    89–90
current generation of patients, 33–34

daily rituals in nursing homes, 91–92
decentralized caregiving networks,
    23–24
decision-makers, 22–24
décor in nursing homes, 95
deference: and control of and within
    nursing home sector, 80–85; and
    humanity as a value, 73–77; and
    moralization of care, 71–72; nursing
    homes as secondary institutions,
    93–99; relational techniques, 86–93;
    and shift in interaction order, xvii;
    spontaneist conception of, 77–80
detachment, 49–50
diagnosis: adjusting to, 12–19; and
    assessment of socio-cultural level,
    50; process of, 7, 9–12, 37–38, 39

diagnostic devices, 9. *See also* clock
test; mini-mental state examination
diary writing, xi–xii
discreditation. *See* loss of credibility
disengagement, 49
disinhibition, 46
diversions, 92, 116–22
Dobbs, Debra, 110
dolls, 123
domestic configurations, 1–4, 21,
24–30
domestic tasks of nursing home
residents, 98
domination, relations of, 132–33
driving, 14, 20, 44, 53–54, 55–56, 58, 59

education levels and discreditation,
50–53
egalitarianism and deference, 74–77
elderliness of patients, 109–10
electric plugs, 96
Elias, Norbert, ix
emergency call buttons, 98
emotional capital, 89
emotional work, 90–91
Ennuyer, Bernard, 99
Estroff, Sue, 108–9
evaluations of nursing home services,
80, 82–85
evidence of good conduct, 48, 49–50

family caregivers: assistance provided
by, 20; Carpentier's study of, xiii–xiv,
7; and discreditation of relatives,
62–64; impact of role on professional
life, 21; and institutional placement
of relatives, 31–32, 63–64
family satisfaction with nursing homes,
82, 91–92
female patients and dolls, 123
female patients' physical appearance,
54–56, 110, 119
financial affairs of patients, 25–26, 31,
64–65

financial position and access to
professional assistance, 20, 22

gender and dementia: females, 54–56,
110, 119, 123; males, 53–54, 55–56
geriatricians, 9, 10
Goffman, Erving, xvi, 5, 49, 75
Gojard, Séverine, 24
Gramain, Agnès, 24
greeting rituals, 108–9
guardianship, 26, 27, 64–65

Hacking, Ian, xvi
Hochschild, Arlie, 90
home configurations, 1–4, 21, 24–30
home model in nursing homes, 96–99
hospital model in nursing homes,
94–96, 98–99
hotel model in nursing homes, 95–96,
97–99
humanization of dementia care, 71–77,
83, 99–100, 130

identity/self, loss and preservation of,
48–50, 123–26
individual autonomy, ix–x, 19–20, 65
institutionalized care, xii–xiii, 30–33,
63–64. *See also* deference
interaction order, x, xiv–xviii
interaction rites, 92–93
interpretation of troubles as dementia-
related, 6, 8–9, 67–70

jokes in reconstitution work, 105–7, 109
Ju/'hoansi people (Botswana), 69
justifying against discreditation, 56–62

Kobelinsky, Carolina, 39

labeling of items, 3, 21
label of "Alzheimer's disease," 11–12
Lamb, Sarah, 131
language and discreditation, 36, 40,
50–51

language issues for migrants, 51, 119–20
latch effect in discreditation process, 47–50
leisure activities, 14–15, 21, 110
lies and credibility, 35, 37
life history binders, 111
life units, 96
little gestures in interactions, xii–xiii
living arrangements and observability of troubles, 6–7
living environment model in nursing homes, 96–99
loneliness, 30
looping effect, xvi
Lopez, Stephen H., 80
loss of autonomy, 19–20
loss of credibility: and alternative ways of interpreting troubles, 67–70; credibility in human interactions, 35–37; effects of, 41–47; factors influencing susceptibility to, 50–56; justifying against, 56–62; latch effect in, 47–50; path toward, 37–41; routinization of, 62–67; and shift in interaction order, xvii
loss of self/identity, 48–50, 123–24
lost talks, 47–50, 56

Mahi, Lara, 35–36
maintenance workers in nursing homes, 97
masculinity and discreditation, 53–54, 55–56
medical interpretation of dementia, x–xi, xvi, 16–17, 67–68
memory consultations, 10–11
memory lapses not related to dementia, 5
memory loss, 39, 124
migrants, 51, 119–20
mini-mental state examination, xi, 11, 45, 51
money matters of patients, 25–26, 31, 64–65

moralization of care, 71–72. *See also* humanization of dementia care
multisensory (Snoezelen) spaces, 30, 112–13

Næss, Anders, 103
Native Americans, 69
neoliberal economic policies and dementia care, 130–31
neurologists, 10
news, patients' interest in, 109–10
nonspeaking patients, 92. *See also* reconstitution
nonverbal deduction, 90
normals (Estroff), 108–9
nurses, 85
nursing aides, xii–xiii, 85, 89, 91, 92, 93
nursing assistants, 85
nursing homes, xii–xiii, 30–33, 63–64. *See also* deference

observability of troubles, 6–8
occupations: formerly held by patients, 49, 110, 112, 114, 115–16, 118, 120–22, 125–26; impact of dementia on, 14, 15–16, 21
odors in nursing homes, 95–96
oligarchic caregiving networks, 23, 24
organization of repairing exchanges: adjusting to diagnosis, 12–19; defined, 4–5; development of caregiving networks, 19–24; diagnostic process, 7, 9–12; and institutionalized care, 30–33; potential patients, 5–9; and shift in interaction order, xvii; trouble management and material configurations, 24–30
organized emotional care, 80

past lives of patients and deference, 92
past lives of patients and reconstitution work, 112–22
peripheral inclusion in discussions, 66–67

pharmaceutical industries' interest in dementia, 9
physical appearance of female patients, 54–56, 110, 119
possessions of institutionalized residents, 31, 32
prevalence of Alzheimer's disease, x
primary and secondary institutions compared, 93–94
professional life. *See* occupations
public policies and dementia, xv, 65, 73, 131

Quebec Department of Health and Social Services, xiii, 73, 82, 93

reconstitution: to act, 115–20; avoiding to maintain order, 120–23; to fill gaps in present interaction, 101–7; and loss and preservation of self, 123–26; and shift in interaction order, xvii–xviii; social content of, 107–11; to understand, 111–15
recordkeeping in nursing homes, 85
recreational activities, 14–15, 21, 100
relational aspect of dementia care work, rewards from, 79–80
relational techniques in deference production, 86–93
relations of domination, 132–33
reminiscence spaces, 30, 109
repairing exchanges. *See* organization of repairing exchanges
representations of dementia, 131–33
Rosenberg, Harriet G., 69

scattered tasks in nursing homes, 97
secondary baby talk, 40
secondary institutions, nursing homes as, 93–99
self-control, ix
self/identity, loss and preservation of, 48–50, 123–26

short-term memory loss, 39
shows of force, 48–50
Skaff, Pamela, xiv
smells in nursing homes, 95–96
Snoezelen (multisensory) spaces, 30, 112–13
social death, 129
social role of living with dementia, 128–30
social status: and deference, 74–77, 83; and diagnosis, 50; and discreditation, 50–53; and institutionalized care, 31; and reconstitution, 110, 113
special attachment of patients to others, 113–14
specialized units in nursing homes, 30
speech difficulties, 92. *See also* reconstitution
Stacey, Clare, 89
successful aging, 131
support bars and handles, 21

tasks in nursing home work, flexibility in, 97
tasks of nursing home residents, 98
time between first troubles and diagnosis, 7
Tocqueville, Alexis de, 76

unit managers, xiii
unwillingness to be institutionalized, 31, 63

vascular dementia, 39, 46–47
verbal communication and discreditation of patients, 40

Weber, Florence, 24
Weber, Max, 99
wheelchairs, alternative names for, 3, 98
whistle-blowers, 22–24
writing in diaries, xi–xii

BAPTISTE BROSSARD is a French sociologist and Lecturer at the Australian National University. He is author of *Why Do We Hurt Ourselves?: Understanding Self-Harm in Social Life.*

CPSIA information can be obtained
at www.ICGtesting.com
Printed in the USA
LVHW051816020819
626320LV00004B/53/P

9 780253 044969